THE SCALE DOES NOT LIE, PEOPLE DO.

Reversing obesity now.
Dr. Nowzaradan takes a closer look at obesity and the essential solutions for the 21th century.

YOUNAN NOWZARADAN M.D.

Medicine is an ever-changing science. The quest for new information and research will broaden our knowledge. Being a doctor and treating the patients who strive to overcome their disease is an art. It is our moral obligation to never give up hope for our patients no matter how difficult the situation may be, because everyone deserves to have quality care, free of prejudice and discrimination.

The Scale Does Not Lie, People Do.
Reversing obesity now. Dr. Nowzaradan takes a closer look at obesity and the essential solutions for the 21th century. First edition.

Houston, TX U.S.A.
Email drnowzaradan@yahoo.com
Ana Karen Castillo Silva IMG. Research assistant.

ISBN (print edition): 978-0-9972252-1-1
ISBN (eBook edition): 978-0-9972252-2-8
Photographs by Jess Ann Aradan Photography.
Illustrations by Jennifer Nowzaradan. www.zaradanfineart.com

If you are battling obesity, you are not alone. Over two hundred million Americans are either overweight or obese. This book is the product of the experiences of an internationally known physician with over four decades of treatment of all forms of obesity. It represents working with individuals that are suffering from obesity and strive to overcome the challenges associated with this disease. The valuable information that you will receive in this book will provide you with some of the best tools which will guide you to make the appropriate changes that are necessary to improve your health, maintain a proper weight, and live a better, healthy and most importantly an enjoyable life.

Many illnesses linked to obesity are known as co-morbid conditions; such as diabetes, high blood pressure, congestive heart failure, respiratory failure, heart attack, stroke and numerous others. Obesity and related illnesses are associated with markedly reduced life expectancy, and it has become a leading cause of preventable death in the United States. It is estimated that each year 300,000 deaths in the United States are attributed to obesity. Obesity is no longer limited to western society. Recent studies show that obesity is a global epidemic. Nearly 2.3 billion people worldwide are either overweight or obese. This represents almost thirty percent of the world's population.

It is estimated that by the year 2030 about 90 percent of the United States population will be either obese or overweight. It is vitally important that we actively seek solutions for this epidemic. By reducing the rate of obesity, we can prevent many comorbid conditions related to obesity and prolong our life expectancy. It is time that we recognize the dangers that we are facing from this epidemic. For many of us the solution to weight management will be our last chance to live.

* * *

July 2025-

Contents

Introduction

As a surgeon, I am blessed with a career that has afforded me on daily basis the ability and opportunity to make a significant difference in people's lives. It is gratifying to witness how a surgical procedure can radically improve someone's quality of life and sometimes save their life.

Weight loss surgery has been particularly rewarding and inspiring. Obesity is linked with higher risks of several health conditions such as high blood pressure, type II diabetes, hyperlipidemia, coronary artery disease, congestive heart failure, obstructive sleep apnea, asthma, respiratory conditions and many forms of cancers. It is impressive to see the resolution of many of these disabling conditions associated with obesity due to weight loss by the surgical intervention. As a result of weight loss surgery, we see elimination or reduction of high blood pressure, diabetes, sleep apnea, congestive heart failure, respiratory difficulties and many other conditions. Additionally, we witness a significant improvement in their quality of life and their emotional wellbeing.

My heart goes out to severely obese individuals who are generally misunderstood, misjudged and invariably shunned by society. Severe obesity is a disease with genetic predisposition; it simply is not a person's choice or their moral failure. It is not entirely due to the lack of discipline and will power. In fact, dieting, exercising and lifestyle modifications would not significantly impact severe obesity and without surgical intervention these individuals will not have a normal life span. Many factors involving severe obesity are simply outside of an individual's control. We should strive to understand their lack of ability to enjoy life, their daily struggles and the humility that they endure.

As a society, we should neither be prejudice nor discriminate against them. We should try to understand that their obesity is not their choice. Severely obese individuals are desperate for care. This segment of our population due to their condition become disabled and economically depressed and considered to be high risk for any medical care. Our response should not be just to eat less and exercise more. Granted the quantity of food consumption will have direct result on the individual's weight gain or loss, but the drive to consume food is what needs to be understood and addressed.

Obesity is a complex, chronic and relapsing metabolic disease as the result of genetic predisposition in a specific environment that is interconnected with groups of many diseases. The metabolic condition of obesity that controls energy balance and calorie expenditure will set the body weight point that it is for most part out of a person's control.

Stigma, bias, prejudice and discrimination against severely obese individuals in our society extends to our healthcare system. Bias and negative attitudes of healthcare providers toward obese individuals that are desperately seeking help, will significantly undermine the outcome of treatment. Inevitably, the quality of care for severely obese individuals falls short of expectations. Sometimes they are denied access to care completely. Imposing weight limits by health care providers and facilities is a good example of such discrimination.

Without a doubt, care of the super morbidly obese, such as 600-pound individuals, requires additional resources and enormous time and effort in comparison to less obese individuals. As a doctor, regardless of how difficult the situation may be, we should never lose hope for any patient. We should understand their disease and their daily struggles. It is our moral obligation to provide them with compassionate quality care, free of prejudice or discrimination. In return, it is truly rewarding and gratifying to witness the transformation of a person that endured a life of misery and suffering into a person who now lives an enjoyable and hopeful life. True happiness is changing the people's lives. We live by each other's happiness not by each other's misery. It is our mission to influence the public as well as the medical community to change bias and negative opinions regarding severely obese individuals.

Obesity is a chronic and progressive disease as a result of a complex metabolic condition that is multifactorial and multidimensional, yet the exact cause of it is not well understood. Obesity at any degree will not only negatively impact our quality of life; but it will shorten our life expectancy and profoundly affect our emotional wellbeing. It is clear that there is no single solution for this complex problem.

Obesity is no longer limited to western society and is becoming a worldwide epidemic. Globally one out of three people are considered obese or overweight, which is nearly one third of the world's population. Despite many advances achieved in the management of obesity, the increased rate of obesity has outpaced effective treatment and its rate continues to increase at an alarming rate.

We should not rely on society to solve the obesity epidemic. Society, by imposing regulations on the food industry is not likely to affect the individual's behavior toward developing healthier eating habits. It is the individual that must make the necessary changes. We should, as individuals, take responsibility to overcome this modern-day epidemic. Our society is based on individual freedom of choice, with freedom comes personal responsibility. It is our personal and moral obligation that we, as individuals, take the initiative to motivate each other for a healthier lifestyle. Management of obesity not only will improve the quality of our lives and prolong our longevity, but it will have a positive effect on our emotional wellbeing. It is our moral obligation of future generations to take the necessary steps to overcome the obesity epidemic in our society. What we do for ourselves as an individual, society cannot do for us. A healthy nation is made of healthy individuals.

In order to achieve our greatest potential in our life we must maintain a positive attitude, possess a desire to improve our life and strive to work hard. We also must have proper knowledge to be able to accomplish this goal. Attitude is everything in our life. We must develop a positive attitude and at the same time we need to understand that life is not always fair and not allow ourselves to become a victim of our life's circumstances. No matter what happens in our life, it matters how we react and respond to it. We must always deal with our emotions in a healthy way and maintain an optimistic and positive attitude. We must learn to develop rational behaviors rather than emotional ones. A positive action combined with positive thinking results in success.

We must also have a desire to change our life for the better. Our life is a reflection of our desires. We live the life we choose. A desire for a better life keeps us motivated and gives us the willingness and determination to discipline ourselves and work hard to achieve our goal in our life. Remember, hard work will have future rewards in our life.

We must also possess the proper knowledge and utilize the right tools to be able to succeed in our life. We cannot know what we don't know. Without proper knowledge we will have no chance to achieve our goals. We must continue to strive to learn, and the more we learn the more we understand how little we know; therefore, we should never stop learning.

It is my objective to inspire and influence you to develop a positive attitude in your life and maintain such a positive attitude no matter how hard things can get in your life. I hope you have the desire to change your life for a better and healthier one and have the willingness and determination to work hard and never give up on reaching your goals in life. We must have goals in life; we must have daily, weekly, monthly, yearly and above all life-time goals.

Food which is necessary for our survival and seems to play a significant role in our life and somehow it controls it. Being overweight or obese not only will impact over physical health negatively, but it will shorten our life expectancy. Obesity also will have a negative effect in our emotional wellbeing. Many of us are faced with frustrations of unsuccessful diets time after time and feel hopeless to lose weight.

Many times, we feel we are different from anyone else and the rules that apply to everyone else do not apply to us. Often, we are looking for a single solution for our problem, but obesity is a complex metabolic condition. Understanding and having proper knowledge of issues involved is essential for proper management of obesity. But first we must disregard and forget all the faulty information, we must separate facts from fiction and start with a clean slate and build information on a solid foundation.

It is time to learn about ourselves, our body, environment, genetics and nutrition. This book is all about providing you with valuable information and giving you the proper tools that you need to succeed in achieving and maintaining a healthy life.

Remember the ingredients to succeed in our life are to have a positive attitude, proper knowledge, desire and willingness to work for it. Imagine yourself thinner, stronger and healthier then strive to achieve this goal.

My objective is to provide you with valuable information and guide you to make the proper changes that are effective for you to lose weight and maintain a healthy lifestyle long term. This plan takes time and persistence, determination, positive attitude, encouragement and willingness to succeed. We do not become this obese or overweight overnight so we should not expect for any changes to occur immediately.

So, let's get started and stay focused on beginning your new life and learn the ingredients that bring a healthy lifestyle to your household.

* * *

Chapter 1
The scale does not lie, people do.

Diane was 342 pounds when I first saw her in my office. During the initial visit it was explained to her that her excessive weight was due to her overeating. For her to lose weight I placed her on a 1200 calorie a day high protein low carb diet and gave her a goal of losing 14 pounds in one month. A month later when she returned for her follow up visit, instead of losing 14 pounds, she had gained 6 pounds while she claimed that she had followed the diet I gave her. I basically told her that she was not being truthful, and she did not follow the diet that I gave her because if she had, she would have lost even more than 14 pounds. The scale is the best lie detector and told me all I needed to know. She really got upset and started crying because I did not believe her.

People like Diane deny their overeating not only to others but to themselves. When they keep lying long enough, they start believing their lies as well as their family but when I don't believe their lies, they become upset and therefore they start crying.

One of the most common eating disorders that is associated with development of obesity is the overconsumption of high calorie foods that easily exceeds 3000 to 4000 calories per day. Yet the individual considers it to be a normal eating habit. Typically, such a false narrative has developed over a long period of time. Many factors such as family dynamic as seen in multigeneration of obesity, or some cultural traditions as well as supersized restaurants and commercial food products, have resulted in misguided eating habits that give the belief and the illusion that their eating habits are normal.

Most often this denial of overeating creates a delusional state that the individual blames their weight problem on many factors other than their eating habits. To them their eating habits are what they should be and magically they have become overweight or obese. They often state "my weight problem is not because of my eating habit, my eating habit is fine" then they add many reasons for their weight problem such as, "I retain fluids", "it is because I don't exercise", "obesity runs in my family" or "it is because of my thyroid problem". Some ladies blame their weight to their menstrual cycle and others to their menopause, some even blame their weight problem on their constipation and the list goes on and on.

The reality is that they refuse to accept the simple fact that their weight is directly related to the number of calories that they consume versus the number of calories they utilize. It is just simple math. The concept of calories in and calories out is actually a very simple one to understand but it seems to be the most difficult one to accept but the reality is that the scale does not lie, people do.

* * *

Chapter 2
Obesity Epidemic

Obesity has become the leading cause of preventable death in the United States. Every year 300,000 deaths are contributed to obesity in America. When BMI is greater than 30 kg/m^2 there is a corresponding associated increased risk of reduced life expectancy and premature death. Research has shown that severe obesity will shorten life expectancy up to 20 years.

Presently 76 percent of the adult population in the United States is considered obese or overweight. It is estimated that by year 2030 this number will rise to nearly 90 percent. 26 percent of the adult population in the United States is considered morbidly obese with a BMI of greater than 50 kg/m^2. This is double the rate of what it was in 1980. Since 1980, the obesity rate has doubled in 70 countries around the world. Globally 2.3 billion people are either obese or overweight. That is nearly one third of the world's population.

In 2015, four million deaths in the world were attributed to obesity. There has been a corresponding increase in rate of type II diabetes mellitus which is directly linked to obesity. For the past few decades, diabetes has been a problem in the US and abroad. Currently, 26 million Americans are affected by type II diabetes mellitus. It is estimated that 79 million people are pre-diabetic and 70 million are not aware of being diabetic.

Childhood and adolescent obesity are also increasing at an alarming rate not only in the United States but worldwide. Recent studies show that over 180 million children globally have a BMI greater than 30 kg/m^2. In the past three decades in the United States the incidence of childhood obesity has tripled, and at the same time the incidence of adolescent obesity has nearly quadrupled. About 32 percent of the children in the United States between the ages of 10 to 17 are overweight and 17 percent are considered obese. The United States had the highest percentages of childhood obesity in 2015.

In the past ten years the military recruit's rejection for weight problems in the United States has jumped from 12 percent to 21 percent. It is predicted that for the first time the longevity of an entire generation will decrease due to obesity. We could witness the sustained drop in our life expectancy in modern times. It is estimated that over the next few decades, life expectancy of an average American could decline by as much as 5 years.

The most practical method of measuring the degree of obesity is defined as the body mass index (BMI). Although there are several more accurate methods of measuring degree of obesity, body mass index is the one most commonly used because of its simplicity. It is calculated weight by kilogram by height in meters squared (kg/m^2). The BMI can be calculated by weight in pounds multiplied by 703 and divided by height in inches twice.

BMI formula: 703 x weight (pound), divided by height (inch) twice. For instance, a person weighing 280 pounds that is 5 feet 10 inches tall the BMI is calculated as follows:

$$280 \times 703 = 196840 \div 70 = 2812 \div 70 = 40.1\ kg/m^2$$

On the following tables find your height and weight and determine your BMI.

	4’9”	4’11”	5’1”	5’3”	5’5”	5’7”	5’9”	5’11	‘6’1”	6’3”
154	33	31	29	27	26	24	23	22	20	19
165	36	33	31	29	28	26	24	23	22	21
176	38	36	33	31	29	28	26	25	23	22
187	40	38	35	33	31	29	28	26	25	24
198	43	40	37	35	33	31	29	28	26	25
209	45	42	40	37	35	33	31	29	28	26
220	48	44	42	39	37	35	33	31	29	28
231	50	47	44	41	39	36	34	32	31	29
243	52	49	46	43	40	38	36	34	32	30
254	55	51	48	45	42	40	38	35	34	32
265	57	53	50	47	44	42	39	37	35	33
276	59	56	52	49	46	43	41	39	37	35
287	62	58	54	51	48	45	42	40	38	36
298	64	60	56	53	50	47	44	42	39	37
309	67	62	58	55	51	48	46	43	41	39
320	69	64	60	57	53	50	47	45	42	40
331	71	67	62	59	55	52	49	46	44	42
342	74	69	65	61	57	54	51	48	45	43
353	76	71	67	63	59	55	52	49	47	44
364	78	73	69	64	61	57	54	51	48	46
375	81	76	71	66	62	59	56	52	50	47
386	83	78	73	68	64	61	57	54	51	48
397	86	80	75	70	66	62	59	56	53	50
408	88	82	77	72	68	64	60	57	54	51
419	90	84	79	74	70	66	62	59	56	53
430	93	87	81	76	72	67	64	60	57	54
441	95	89	83	78	73	69	65	62	58	55
452	98	91	85	80	75	71	67	63	60	57
463	100	93	87	82	77	73	69	65	61	58

- BMI 19 to 24.9 – Healthy Weight
- BMI 25 to 29.9 – Overweight
- BMI 30 to 34.99 – Obese - Class I obesity
- BMI 35 to 39.9 – Severely obese - Class II obesity
- BMI 40 and up – Morbidly obese - Class III obesity

Healthy weight (lbs.) for BMI 18-25 kg/m^2

BMI Height	18	19	20	21	22	23	24	25
5’	92	97	102	108	113	118	123	128
5’1’’	95	101	106	111	116	122	127	132
5’2’’	98	104	109	115	120	126	131	137
5’3’’	102	107	113	119	124	130	135	141
5’4’’	105	111	117	122	128	134	140	146
5’5’’	108	114	120	126	132	138	144	150
5’6’’	112	118	124	130	136	143	149	155
5’7’’	115	121	128	134	140	147	153	160
5’8’’	118	125	132	138	145	151	158	164
5’9’’	122	129	135	142	149	156	163	169
5’10’’	125	132	139	146	153	160	167	174
5’11’’	129	136	143	151	158	165	172	179
6’	133	140	147	155	162	170	177	184
6’1’’	136	144	152	159	167	174	182	190
6’2’’	140	148	156	164	171	179	187	195
6’3’’	144	152	160	168	176	184	192	200
6’4’’	148	156	164	173	181	189	197	205

The changes in the modern-day lifestyle and permissive food environment as well as our dietary habits have been partially responsible for the global significant increased rate of obesity. Despite widespread anti-obesity campaigns with preventive strategies and an abundance of treatment modalities for obesity, its rate has outpaced its effective treatment and continues to increase at an alarming rate. The prevalence of obesity is not only seen in Western society but in the entire world, it has reached to an epidemic level.

Sadly, national and global anti-obesity campaigns and obesity preventing strategies remain inefficient in reducing the rate of obesity. It is estimated in the United States by the year 2030 nearly 90 percent of Americans will be obese or overweight. As a matter of fact, health care reform and comprehensive strategies about healthy diet and physical activity have not impacted the rapidly escalating rate of obesity, mostly because they fail to address the common underlying causes.

The economic burden of obesity on society has given the society a cause to impose regulations on freedom of choice regarding eating habits. Many governments around the world are imposing regulatory interventions against calorie concentrated high sugar content food items and beverages. They are imposing high taxation on these food items and limiting the size of beverages and preventing measures against advertising as well as mandating warning labels. Such measures are not likely going to change individual behaviors toward their eating habits. In the past utilizing similar regulations regarding alcohol and tobacco use has been proven to be ineffective. Such regulations are not only against our nature, removing discretion and limiting personal freedom of choice but they also fail to address the common underlying causes as well.

After 5,000 to 6,000 years that we as human beings have been in existence, we still have no consensus of opinion regarding what constitutes healthy eating habits. After all, with over 2,000 different and contradicting weight loss diets and over hundreds of weight loss medications and remedies and several surgical treatments of obesity, we are creating an array of contradictory and confusing choices that contribute to the failure effective weight loss effort. So far obesity rate has outpaced its ineffective treatment and preventive measures, and its trend continues to increase in an alarming rate.

Anti-obesity campaigns and preventative strategies should not be negative. We should neither stigmatize obese individuals nor demonize food industry. Our message should be positive but much more than eat less and exercise more.

In order to achieve our greatest potential in life we must have four essential characteristics. First, we must have a positive and correct **attitude**. Attitude is everything in our life. It is our emotions and our beliefs that shape our behavior and our objective in life, it gives meaning and purpose to our life. No matter what the circumstances are in our life we must shape our attitude to be positive and optimistic at all times. Our attitude not only affects us, but it will affect how others interact with us as well. We must understand that our life has ups and downs. Where there is success there will be failure. Where there is a gain there will be a loss. When there is a pleasure there will be pain. When there is laughter there will be crying. Where there is happiness there will be sadness. Where there is sunshine there will be rain. We need to understand that life can be unfair at times, we must change the way we look at things in our life. A positive attitude will not allow us to become victim of circumstances. No matter what happens is in our life it matters how we react to it, if we keep our face to sunshine the dark shadow will always be behind us. A positive attitude is essential for us to succeed in our life, without the right attitude we will never succeed in our life. The fact is that we can change our attitude in our life and the way we look at the things in our life and if we do, the things in our life will change too.

Second, we must have **desire** to change our life for the better. Our life reflects our desires. We live the life we choose. Desire is the one that will set our goals in our life; we must have goals in our life to be able to succeed.

The third characteristic in life is our **willingness** to work hard, discipline ourselves to pay the price, and work hard to achieve our goals.

The fourth characteristic in our life is **knowledge**. Having proper knowledge is a tool that gives us the road map to success, without proper knowledge it looks like we need to go somewhere but don't know where and will not ever get there. We need to continue to learn and expand our knowledge and the more we learn the more we understand how little we know.

In order to achieve our greatest potential in our life we must have all four characteristics. Those four characteristics of **attitude**, **desire**, **willingness** and **knowledge** are a chain that cannot have a missing link. If we have the right attitude but we have no desire to change our life, we will not succeed. If we have the right attitude and desire to change our life for the better, but no willingness to work hard to achieve this, we will not get there. If we have the right attitude and desire to change our life and willingness to work hard but lacking proper knowledge we will not succeed.

Society instead of imposing rules and regulations on personal freedom of choice and behavior should attempt to build the four characteristics necessary to achieve our greatest potential in life.

It is my hope and objective to inspire you to develop all four characteristics in your life to succeed in achieving a healthy lifestyle, and proper knowledge that will provide you with long-term success.

We must have dreams in our life because our life is the reflection of our dreams. We must pay the price, work hard, meet the challenges, and never quit to make our dreams come true. A dream needs a goal in our life because a dream without a goal is just a dream. We must have a daily, weekly, monthly, yearly goal and above all a lifetime goal. Life can be tough, but we must find someone to help us through life. We must know that life is not fair, and we will often fail but we must have the will to succeed and never ever give up.

We must discipline ourselves to work hard every day and not to be afraid to go to bed late and still get up early the next day. Little things in life matter, if we can't do the little things right, we won't be able to do the big things right. Start every day with a task and end the day with a task completed and tomorrow will be a better day.

We must respect everyone but first have a sense of self-respect and sense of pride in what we do. We must learn to lift ourselves up but in the meantime lift others up with us. We must change our life for the better, and at the same time the life of others. We must live by each other's happiness.

We must have a positive influence on the lives of others and be the one who inspires them. Remember others will measure us by the size of our hearts and not by who we are. We must understand the meaning of our life. This life is not about what we take when we leave this world; it is about what we leave behind. Remember the future is in our hands. We live the life we choose and the choices we make in our life will have future consequences.

* * *

Chapter 3
Economic impact of obesity

Obesity and related illnesses pose a major health problem and significant economic burden to every society around the world and is becoming a global phenomenon.

Obesity increases the risk of multiple diseases such as high blood pressure, type 2 diabetes, sleep apnea, coronary artery disease and certain type of cancers. There is increased health care cost associated with obesity both in terms of diagnosis as well as treatment. Medical cost among obese adults are 42 percent higher than individuals with normal weight. The annual cost of obesity and its related illnesses in the United States exceeds 414 billion dollars. This is an excess of 21 percent of annual total healthcare cost. With the rapid increase rate of obesity this cost is estimated to escalate over 586 billion dollars by the year 2023. The cost of treatment of cardiovascular disease such as high blood pressure, coronary artery disease and stroke is estimated to be 315.8 billion dollars per year. The cost associated with treatment of type 2 diabetes is over 245 billion dollars annually. Eighty percent of people with type 2 diabetes are considered obese. The economic burden of obesity in society is much more than can meet the eyes. The indirect ripple effect of obesity on the economy is difficult to estimate.

The negative impact of obesity in the workplace is not only related to the increased cost of insurance in obese individuals due to higher utilization of diagnostic and therapeutic services, but it is also related to loss of productivity. This is due to illnesses requiring short term or long-term disability or leaving the work force due to permanent disability or death. This loss of productivity in the workplace is not limited to absenteeism from work but also the loss of productivity caused by mobility deficits, daytime sleepiness, loss of concentration or reduced cognitive ability and medication side effects, which results in increased risk of injuries as well.

Obesity has also impacted the healthcare system negatively. Hospitals and health care facilities are required to purchase expensive specialized equipment to accommodate heavier patients such as larger blood pressure cuffs, larger wheelchairs and stretchers, bariatric hospital beds, larger shower facilities with reinforced toilets to accommodate large bodies. The cost increases due to the purchase of larger capacity CT SCAN, X-ray equipment and MRI with higher weight limits. It also requires hiring additional employees to provide transportation. Emergency response team in order to transport larger and overweight patients requires specialized oversized bariatric equipment and several more personnel. This has increased healthcare costs tremendously.

Obese patients when hospitalized require a longer length of stay compared to normal weight patients. Additionally, if they require surgery they are at a higher risk of postoperative complications.

Along with the increased rate of severe obesity and related illnesses, there is an increased rate of disability claims which qualifies them to receive free medical care. There is a substantial cost involved in providing severe obese individuals with monthly disability income as well as medical supplies and equipment such as canes, walkers, shower chairs, hospital beds, wheelchairs and even motorized scooters. In some cases, they are also provided with one or more paid care giver to help them in activities of daily living, which is often a member of the family or a friend. Usually a disabled obese individual is a source of financial support to the entire family and household.

Their severe obesity in many cases may not be individual's choice and the circumstances that lead to their obesity may simply be outside of their control, but willingness to overcome obesity remains their choice. Receiving disability benefits is highly addictive. In many cases treatment of food addiction and obesity is far less challenging than giving up free social disability benefits. Our society by being compassionate and providing disability benefits to morbidly obese individuals is creating an unintended consequence by proliferating entitlement attitude that discourages motivation and willingness to overcome obesity, because of fear of losing disability benefits.

* * *

Chapter 4
Understanding our dietary habits

Food is necessary for survival. It plays a significant role in our life. Hunger and the desire to eat are basic survival instincts in humans as well as other species. A close look at the dietary habits of humans in comparison to other species shows some significant differences. Animals and other species possess a powerful instinct to choose and recognize proper food that is uniform and similar in all species. For example, cows worldwide eat grass. All penguins eat krill, squid and fish. Pandas eat the stems of bamboo; therefore, they must live in an environment where bamboo can grow. Most all animals and other species choose their food by instinct unlike humans. We as humans do not have this instinct, we must use our discretion and judgment to make our food choices. This phenomenon is contrary to the theory of evolution.

If we evolved from primates as a successive generation, the inheritable characteristics of biological property should have been passed on to us. We should be able to recognize our food source by instinct, but we don't, this is clearly contradictory to the theory of evolution. We as humans have no consensus or opinion as to what the proper food choices are. Every culture and society worldwide have formulated different food choices that are vastly different. Many cultures in the Far East consider eating live insects, worms, snakes, dogs and monkey's brains to be their food choices. Here in America none of these choices are considered appropriate. No matter how perfect our discretions or choices for food are, they will never match or be as perfect as animal instincts. It is speculated that we as human beings have been in existence on earth for 5,000 to 6,000 years yet we have not come to a uniform consensus of opinion regarding what constitutes proper food choices.

Another significant difference in our dietary habits when compared to other species is the regulatory mechanism of food intake. Stability of body weight and its composition over a long period requires that the energy intake from food sources and energy expenditure to be balanced. The regulatory mechanism of food intake and dietary balance in most other species and animals is more efficient than human being. Their efficient mechanism of food intake prevents them from overeating. It only allows them to eat enough to survive. They do not overeat which is why we don't see obesity in animals or other species.

Human beings from newborn through infancy has an efficient regulatory mechanism for food intake that prevents them overeating. As we mature, the regulatory mechanism fades away. As adolescents this mechanism begins to be controlled by judgment and discretion. These judgments and discretions are influenced by environmental factors, emotions, psychological and genetic factors. Imbalances in any of these areas lead to overeating and obesity. We do not witness this in animals. For example, if you leave a cow with an abundant supply of grass it will only eat a sufficient amount and will not overeat. Likewise, a lion or tiger will hunt and kill their prey and will eat the proper amount and walk away leaving the remainder behind. This efficiency of their regulatory mechanism for food intake prevents them from overeating and therefore we don't see obese lions or tigers.

Based on the differences between our eating habits when compared with other species it clearly indicates that the evolution theory is not applicable. It is logical to assume that we are created by an intelligent design rather than a by-product of evolution. We are given discretion and freedom to choose our food rather than having instinct. Our dietary habits are linked to our longevity. Our genetic predisposition and our dietary habits are linked together. When we are born the end of life event is programmed in our genes. We all have an expiration date that is linked to our eating habits and genetic predisposition. It is our nature by design that we choose what to eat, how much and how often.

Genetic predisposition can lead to cardiovascular disease, high blood pressure, stroke, heart attack, cancer, diabetes, obesity and all these related illnesses are linked to our inefficient dietary habits by design.

Significant changes have been made to lifestyle habits over the past one hundred years. As the world modernized, this created a fast-paced lifestyle with limited time and the inability to devote and prepare nutritional meals which met our dietary requirements. As result, we have shifted our discretion of making food choices to the food industry. The food industry stepped up to fill this void. They created food choices which have been chemically altered for taste and ease of digestion. This has opened the door to overconsumption of food and food addiction.

As a result, we witnessed a permissive environment which began to make over consumption of food the norm. Societal accommodations for obesity have been mandated. Obesity is now a worldwide epidemic which is persistently and steadily growing. It is important to understand that our longevity in life is highly linked to our dietary habits. These habits are left to our discretion and choices which can be highly inefficient and harmful to our well-being.

In order to break free from allowing the food industry to influence our discretion we must garner proper knowledge and understanding of science, physiology and metabolism to make healthy food choices. We as humans are the most intelligent species in the world and have a great ability to build on tangible knowledge from one generation to the next. We have built the most amazing buildings, machinery and equipment. At the same time, we are incapable to build on intangible knowledge from one generation to the next; the basic logical human behavior and ethic in certain aspects has not significantly changed in the past 5000-6000 years. We have not been able to build on the practical knowledge of nutrition and dietary habits as well.

The medical professionals have considered obesity to be a behavioral and moral failure and formed bias and stigma against obese individuals for the longest time. Physicians were trained inadequately in obesity medicine and did nothing to treat obesity but to recommend eat less and exercise more. For the past 20 years obesity medicine has become a subspecialty leaving a gap in training physicians to properly understand that obesity is a disease and that many factors involving in this disease are simply outside of individual's control and it is not entirely due to lack of discipline or will power.

Obesity is a complex, chronic relapsing metabolic disease as result of genetic predisposition in a specific environment that is interconnected to a group of illnesses. Obesity is due to interaction of multiple genes that control composition of many hormones that effect energy balance, food intake and calorie consumption that will determine body weight set point. The most effective modality of the treatment of obesity is weight loss surgery that causes hormonal alteration that will change energy balance to a lower weight set point. However, the genetic predisposition of obesity will gradually reverse the hormonal change to the original state and higher body set point.

There are over 2,000 different and contradictory weight loss diets, hundreds of weight loss medications and remedies. This array of contradicting and confusing choices only makes it more difficult to choose the right path and nearly makes it impossible to succeed in a weight loss journey.

Over the years we have formed habits and opinions regarding our eating habits. Some of these are based on erroneous circulating opinions that have become basis of the foundation over our current knowledge. Building on such faulty foundations will inevitably collapse. We cannot know what we do not know. The more we learn the more we understand how little we know; therefore, we should be humble and keep an open mind and forget what we know. Begin with a fresh start and build on a foundation based on proven scientific facts.

This book will provide you with useful information based upon scientific evidence of the human anatomy and physiology that will give you the ability to improve your discretion regarding your dietary habits and provide you with thc proper tools to achieve a healthy lifestyle.

* * *

Chapter 5
Understanding causes of obesity

Obesity is defined as a condition of excessive fat accumulation in the body to the extent that well-being is adversely affected. It is a direct result of positive and imbalance of daily calorie intake from the food and daily calorie expenditure. This positive calorie intake over a period of time will result in excess calories to be stored in the body in the form of fat and cause obesity. Stability of our body weight and its composition over a long period of time requires that energy intake from the food sources and energy expenditure to be balanced. The regulatory mechanism of food intake in our early stages of life maintains an efficient balance so newborn and a child will not overeat. As we grow up this efficiency gradually fades away. When adolescent age is reached, it gradually shifts to our choice and discretion to make food choice. Our adulthood weight will be the result of the dietary habits developed during adolescent and teenage years.

Many factors affect our daily food intake, metabolism and calorie expenditure. If calorie intake on a daily basis exceeds our calorie expenditure, we will be prone to become obese or overweight. Obesity is a complex metabolic condition that is multifactorial and multidimensional. Our metabolism is the result of interactions of many hormones in our body. These hormones are due to multiple inheritable genes in our body. Genetic factors that cause obesity play a role in more than 85 percent of the cases. Genetic predisposition of obesity is in our DNA. More often genetic predisposition of obesity is due to the interaction of multiple genes that control several hormones in the gastrointestinal system as well as peripheral hormones. Diabetic and obesity genes are dominant genes so the incidence of obesity and related illnesses will increase with every next generation. For the past 5,000 to 6,000 years those genes are being passed onto the next generations, so the incidence of obesity and diabetes will continue to rise in every next generation.

In the past few decades, the obesity rate has increased rapidly all over the world. Since 1980, the rate of obesity has doubled in 70 countries around the world. Globally 2.3 billion people are either obese or overweight. It is estimated by 2030 nearly 90 percent of Americans will be obese or overweight. Such a rapid increase in the rate of obesity is more than genetic factors can explain.

Aside from the genes that are in our DNA there are many inheritable genes that are not in our DNA. These genes remain dormant in our body. Biological regulatory system throughout our body is responsive to environmental factors that can modify these hereditary gene expressions without altering our DNA sequence. This response is called epigenetic modification. Many human diseases including obesity, type II diabetes, cancer and arteriosclerosis can be explained by epigenetic and exogenous factors that cause obesity.

One example of epigenetic modification in development of disease is the infection by Epstein-Barr virus that cause infectious mononucleosis. In certain individuals this causes a chronic disease known as chronic fatigue syndrome, but also this virus in certain individuals along with dietary habits and environmental factors can interact with human genoma and activate many autoimmune diseases such as lupus, multiple sclerosis, rheumatoid arthritis, idiopathic juvenile arthritis, inflammatory bowel disease, type I diabetes and celiac disease.

It is important to understand that our genetic predisposition of obesity and metabolism are endogenous causes of obesity that are beyond our control. However, the environmental changes of epigenetic or exogenous causes of obesity are in our control and can be altered by behavior modification and lifestyle changes.

So, it is important to understand that anti-obesity campaign and prevention strategies can only affect the epigenetic factor of obesity and do not address the common underlying causes of obesity.

No doubt over the past few decades significant changes have happened to modern lifestyle. Along with the increase of personal and global economic growth, it is noted that there has been a corresponding increase rate of obesity. Global industrial and agricultural advancements have created a major shift in the availability of the low-cost global food supply that is making food affordable. Global growth of supermarkets and fast food restaurants are corresponding with overconsumption of food. The food industry is a competitive market that is constantly modifying and chemically altering the food so that it not only digests rapidly but develops an addictive taste. Food products are increasingly becoming calorie dense with a high carbohydrate, sugar and fat content. Energy drinks with high sugar content are widely available. Currently inexpensive and highly processed and chemically engineered foods are widely available in many countries around the world.

It is human nature that we use our discretion regarding food choices as well as frequency and amount of food we eat. However, with modern lifestyle changes, we have shifted our discretion to the food industry that has opened the door for overconsumption of high calorie food.

The economic burden that obesity placed on society, has given the society the necessity to impose regulations on personal freedom of choice. Society by imposing taxation, requiring warning signs on the food label and limiting the size of beverages, is not likely going to change individual's behavior toward their eating habits.

Automated environment of modern life has brought technological advancement in transportation and wide spreading elevators and escalators that reduces the need for any physical activity. Automated factory and industries have reduced or eliminated the need for manual labor. The invention of digital devices and phones has increased sedentary lifestyle, this leaves very little or no time for personal health and exercise.

An additional factor affecting our epigenetic is that the modern lifestyle tends to cause more stressful circumstances that create stress related eating habits that promotes obesity.

Many emotional and psychological conditions result in seeking food for comfort. Depression can be a trigger point for overeating and weight gain or even obesity. Food comfort reduces the stress response. Modern day lifestyle is more prone to stressful situations. Post-traumatic stress disorder is associated with an increased desire to eat. Food addiction is an addictive personality that allows the person to abuse food in similar manner as alcohol, tobacco or even drugs that can be the cause of obesity.

All these factors in the past four decades cannot adequately explain worldwide rapid escalating rate of obesity. One overlooked factor that recent research has shown as a major shift and a key factor in proliferation of obesity is the role of gastrointestinal microbiota.

Our body hosts numerous live microorganisms in our gastrointestinal tract. These are harmless microbes that are necessary for our survival. These microorganisms are essential for healthy function of our digestive system, immune response and metabolic process. Colonization of human gastrointestinal tract starts in vitro and continues at birth.

As time goes on additional microorganisms are acquired in our system. As the number of these microbes increases our gastrointestinal function improves and we will be able to handle and digest different food items. The baby's microorganisms are generally similar to their mothers. Babies that are delivered vaginally have a greater number of microbes than those delivered by cesarean section.

These microorganisms are also known as gut microbiota. Human gastrointestinal microbes impact host metabolism by production of various proteins, including hormones and neurotransmitters that can activate signaling pathways in the gut and also enter the circulation, resulting in effect on insulin resistance, inflammation and deposition of energy in fat stores. Also, gut microbiota produces short-chain fatty acids that result in fat deposition.

Gastrointestinal microbiota aside from their function in the digestive system and developing digestive enzymes, are an important factor in developing the framework of our immune system. Exposure to these harmless bacteria results in development of multiple antibodies that build our immune system. In addition, the gut bacteria play a significant role in our metabolism and food intake. This symbiotic relationship of body and gut microorganisms is such that we will provide their food that is necessary for their existence. The gut bacteria will affect absorption of food at pathway of insulin secretion as well as insulin resistance and the secretion off Ghrelin and our drive to eat, and that is how they influence our body weight.

The gut bacteria act as separate endocrine organ that affect our choices of food intake and play a significant role in developing obesity, metabolic syndrome, type II diabetes and cardiovascular disease. With the world-wide changes we have made in our environment, such as widespread use of chemicals, pesticides, and the use of many different medications as well as antibiotics we have altered and shifted the colonization of the gut microbiota. This microbial shift is known as dysbiosis of the gastrointestinal microbiota. For the past several decades it seems that such changes in colonization of gastrointestinal microbiota have adversely affected our metabolism. Looking at history of how we have dealt with the bacteria in the past has shown us that we have no clue as to how the microbial population has altered their characteristics to continue affecting our life.

The history of world is intertwined with the impact of infectious diseases on the world population. In the year 370 BC Hippocrates wrote about the spread of disease by means of air, water and places. He made the association between climate, diet and living conditions. In the 1500s the theory of the germs and their transmission by means of direct contact and being airborne was introduced. By the 1600s the development of the microscope allowed visualization of microorganisms for the first time. In the 1800s we developed the knowledge of cultivation and identification of bacteria and viruses. Vaccines and antibiotics were developed to control and prevent some infectious diseases.

Pasteurization was another important breakthrough in the reduction of the infectious diseases. The importance of nutrition was appreciated for its impact on the infectious diseases. In the 20th century breakthrough with pharmacotherapy and antibiotics was made into the infectious disease armamentarium. Despite all the progress we have made in dealing with infectious diseases, when we eradicate a disease another appears. We have been able to control leprosy, plague, syphilis, smallpox, Cholera, yellow fever, typhoid fever and many other infectious diseases. New demographics in international traveling have dramatically changed gut microbiota. In 1976, Ebola virus was first identified in Africa. Since then, the world health organization has reported a total of 24 outbreaks of this deadly disease. Now we are dealing with a new emerging infectious disease which we have no clue to how the new agents have appeared. Human immunodeficiency virus (HIV), for the first time was identified in 1981. Presently HIV is a leading cause of death in Africa and fourth leading cause of death in the world.

It appears that we are dealing with a new frontier of microorganisms which we thought had a symbiotic relationship with our body and was necessary for our gastrointestinal function and immune system, but instead now it is invoking obesity, type II diabetes and cardiovascular disease and in fact shortening our longevity. Now it is becoming clearer that in the past few decades what we thought was the only cause of the obesity epidemic was the availability of fast and processed food, but indeed is due to dysbiosis of our gastrointestinal microbiota as well. Although quite complex, there is a new emerging clarity about the association of the development of obesity, metabolic disorder, the risk of type II diabetes and cardiovascular disease with dysbiotic gut microbiota that not only alter our metabolism but also influences our drive for food intake and affect our calorie expenditure.

A promising future treatment of obesity may be pharmaceuticals that will be able to alter gastrointestinal microbial flora to control our eating habits and maintain a healthy weight. Recent studies show that Metformin, the most commonly prescribed medication for diabetes changes gastrointestinal bacterial function and increases the ability to create helpful short chain fatty acids that lower the blood sugar. The newer drugs hopefully will be able to treat metabolic disease, diabetes and obesity.

Recent research has shown that intestinal microbiota from a lean donor successfully changes some of the composition of the gut microbiota of obese individuals. This is possibly a positive step forward for the treatment of obesity.

In summary, in the past few decades multiple factors have come together to create the perfect storm for obesity pandemic. Genetic predisposition of obesity with epigenetic modifications in response to environmental factors play an important role in the global obesity epidemic. Development of worldwide abundant food supply that is inexpensive and calorie concentrated along with modern lifestyle that replaces and eliminates the need for physical activity, have been cofactors in this phenomenon. A key factor has been dysbiosis of the gastrointestinal microbiota. This has been the result of widespread chemical use in our daily life and agricultural pesticides, as well as use of many new medications and antibiotics and changes of our dietary habits. These shifts in our gastrointestinal microbial population have resulted in metabolic changes that control our food intake and energy expenditure and are the prime cause of obesity epidemic, type II diabetes and cardiovascular diseases.

Although there is no single solution for this complex problem, the promising of new treatment to prevent obesity epidemic may come in the form of pharmaceutical agents, or gastrointestinal microbiota transplantation of a lean person that may be beneficial in altering the microflora of gastrointestinal tract and normalize our food intake. But nevertheless, a large-scale public education regarding healthy eating habits with lifestyle changes, as well as development of sense of personal responsibility and self-motivation will be far more beneficial than imposing regulations on the food industry and restricting personal freedom of choice.

* * *

Chapter 6
Diseases associated with obesity

Obesity causes multiple health related issues that are known as comorbid conditions. They are called this because they can and will result in an early death. The profound effect of obesity on cardiovascular, liver and respiratory systems is a major cause of premature death. Obesity is a significant factor in the development of type 2 diabetes and insulin resistance even in children and adolescent.

Obesity also causes hyperlipidemia and metabolic syndrome; it is a major cause of obstructive sleep apnea and respiratory insufficiency. It also aggravates many respiratory illnesses such as asthma. Obesity related habitual snoring and poor quality of sleep contribute to daytime sleepiness, loss of productivity, poor brain function and impaired judgment. The effect of obesity on kidney function and the urinary system causes a variety of symptoms, including recurrent urinary tract infections and urinary incontinence.

Increased body fat acts as an endocrine organ that produces multiple inflammatory molecules that affect and interact with hormones such as corticosteroid, estrogen and insulin. It releases multiple by-products that can cause premature tissue aging and age-related illnesses. Accelerated tissue aging is associated with the development of age-related diseases occurring at a markedly younger age.

The effect of obesity on the reproductive system is a major cause of infertility both in male and female. Obesity is also known to be the contributing factor for the development of polycystic ovarian syndrome (PCOS) in females.

Inflammatory joint disease as well as degenerative joint disease and gout are more common in obese individuals. Obesity is known to be a major cause of gastroesophageal reflux disease.

Many cancers, including breast, colorectal, endometrium, esophagus, gallbladder, kidney, pancreas, and thyroid are linked to obesity. The effect of obesity on the liver is known as fatty infiltration of the liver that is known to cause liver failure, cirrhosis of the liver and potential to develop liver cancer.

In many cases idiopathic intracranial pressure known as pseudotumor cerebri is linked to obesity. Increased intra-abdominal fat and adipose tissue is associated with decreased brain function. Obesity is associated with increased risk of thromboembolism (blood clot) and increased risk of development of pulmonary embolism that can be associated with high risk of mortality. Obesity increases the risk of anesthesia, surgical risk, postsurgical complications and results in increased length of hospital stays. Depression and mental health problems are more common in obese individuals.

Social bias and discrimination, excess sweating, body odor and poor personal hygiene are factors that affect quality of life and emotional well-being of obese persons.

Effective treatment of obesity in many cases can reduce or eliminate most of comorbid conditions associated with obesity, that not only improve quality of life but prolongs life expectancy.

Effect of Obesity on Cardiovascular System

The dramatic effect of obesity on the cardiovascular system is one of the major causes of premature death. The heart is an organ that pumps blood into our blood vessels. The right side of the heart pumps the blood into the lungs for oxygenation, the blood then returns to the left side of the heart, which will be pumped into the arteries to circulate throughout our entire body. The blood carries oxygen and nutrients to the cells in our body.

Obesity increases the resistance to the blood flow due to the excess fatty tissue makes it harder for the blood to pass through the blood vessels. Obesity is associated with high blood pressure. Hormonal changes in the body as a result of obesity along with increased resistance to blood flow lead to high blood pressure, also called hypertension. Increased blood pressure exerts a major strain on the left side of the heart. This strain causes the heart to become enlarged and the heart valves weaken and fail to function properly. This condition is called "Ventricular Hypertrophy". Every obese individual suffers from a variable degree of ventricular hypertrophy. This condition may be well tolerated in its early stages, but over time it worsens and leads to congestive heart failure that severely affects a person's functional capacity. Congestive heart failure results in fluid buildup in the tissue, legs and lungs. This build-up of fluid causes shortness of breath and inability to perform any physical activity. Additionally, obesity results in structural changes in the heart muscle that is known as "cardiomyopathy" resulting in significant heart flutters, irregular heartbeats and sudden death.

Obesity also causes right heart failure known as "pulmonary hypertension". This is a very debilitating disease that causes extreme shortness of breath, dizziness, swelling of the feet and legs. Also known as "cor-pulmonale" and it is associated with syncope, where a person falls down and loses consciousness. Pulmonary hypertension is associated with marked decreased tolerance of physical activity and the person is unable to lay down flat. This condition leads to cardiac arrest and premature death.

The dramatic effect of obesity on the cardiovascular system is augmented by the parallel negative effect on the other organs especially the respiratory system. This multi-organ effect of obesity poses a major risk for general anesthesia and sudden death. All these negative effects create a major concern with any surgical intervention that requires general anesthesia in obese individuals due to the increased risk of death.

The effect of obesity on blood vessels when combined with high blood pressure causes structural changes in the blood vessels which promotes premature hardening of the arteries known as "arteriosclerosis". The effect of arteriosclerosis of the coronary arteries causes premature heart attacks and when it affects the neck and brain vessels it results in stroke and transient ischemic attacks, organic brain syndrome and dementia.

The effect of high blood pressure on kidneys results in chronic kidney disease and renal failure that is a major cause of renal dialysis.

High blood pressure causes structural changes in the walls of the blood vessels and results in aneurysm (ballooning of blood vessels). An aneurysm is a major risk factor in blood clot formation, rupturing of blood vessels and fatal hemorrhage.

The effect of obesity, high blood pressure, hardening of arteries, atherosclerosis (cholesterol building up on the walls of the arteries) are major contributors of poor circulation, which is one of the most common causes of amputation and loss of limbs.

Obesity also affects the venous system in our body. It can cause venous stasis, varicose veins and blood clot formation known as "deep venous thrombosis" (DVT). These venous system problems cause a migration of a blood clot into the right heart and lodge in the pulmonary vessels of the lung. This clot causes serious disruption of blood return to left side of the heart, that disrupts oxygenation and can result in sudden death. Obese individuals are at high risk of development of DVT and pulmonary embolism with any surgical procedure. Each year over one hundred thousand deaths are contributed to pulmonary embolism. Ten percent of the individuals affected by pulmonary embolism will not make it to the hospital alive.

Effect of Obesity on the Lungs and Respiratory System

One of the profound effects of obesity on the respiratory system is the development of “hypoventilation syndrome”. This syndrome is caused by the accumulation of fatty tissue surrounding the respiratory muscles. These muscles aids in moving air in and out of the lungs. This fatty tissue build-up places a heavy weight on the chest and combined with increased intra-abdominal pressure severely limits the lung’s ability to expand and contract. Also, the accumulation of fat in the abdomen markedly elevates the diaphragm reducing the lung’s capacity and ability to breath. Restriction of the lung function will result in decreased oxygen saturation and increased carbon dioxide (CO_2) in the blood. As result person will always feel tired or out of breath and experience daytime sleepiness and develop mental sluggishness.

Another problem with increased carbon dioxide in the blood is a condition known as CO_2 narcosis. CO_2 narcosis with hypoventilation syndrome is associated with high risk of respiratory failure, when a person is lying flat that can lead to loss of consciousness and sudden death. This is known as supine death syndrome that is prevalent among obese individuals. Hypoventilation syndrome increases the risk of premature coronary artery disease, heart attacks, strokes and cerebrovascular accident. Obesity aggravates asthma and reactive airway disease. The effect of obesity on the lung and cardiovascular system causes pulmonary hypertension, which is a significantly debilitating disease that causes severe limitation of physical activity and a high rate of premature death.

The combined effect of obesity on the cardiovascular system causes a major concern placing these obese individuals at a very high risk for general anesthesia. Administering general anesthesia may result in sudden death. Frequently the person experiences respiratory failure requiring prolonged ventilator support and the need for placement of a tracheostomy that is associated with increased risk for complications and a high rate of premature death. Due to the complications associated with the effects of obesity on the respiratory and cardiovascular systems, these obese individuals inevitably endure prolonged hospitalization. This will require an increase in hours of care followed by intensive physical rehabilitation which can take months to accomplish. Thus, obesity imposes a significant financial burden on our society and the health care system.

One of the most serious respiratory consequences of obesity is obstructive sleep apnea. Obesity is a major cause of the development of obstructive sleep apnea. This obstruction is due to increases in upper airway soft tissue resistance. During sleep, muscle tone relaxes which results in snoring, breathing becomes shallow and as it progresses the upper airway completely blocks the flow of air to the lungs. This is called apnea. Apnea causes a drop in the oxygen level and increases carbon dioxide in the circulating blood. This wakes the person up and they will start breathing with a choking sound and the person will fall readily back to sleep, they will have no recollection of this event. This phenomenon repeats continuously throughout sleep. The individuals with sleep apnea are rarely aware of their difficulty of breathing. Often sleep apnea is only recognized as a problem by others witnessing an episode of apnea.

Sleep disturbance pattern prevents deep sleep and results in ineffective sleep and poor resting. Often the person wakes up in the morning with a dry mouth and sore throat. Morning headaches, being tired, having low energy, being drowsy, poor concentration ability and being sleepy all day are some of the symptoms of sleep apnea. It is not unusual for the person to fall asleep at work and even while driving. Sleep apnea increases the risk of automobile accidents and errors in daily job performance. Men are twice as likely as women to be affected by obstructive sleep apnea. Sleep apnea increases risks of cardiovascular problems such as high blood pressure, heart attack and stroke. To manage the effects of sleep apnea, doctors prescribe the use of a continuous positive pressure machine called CPAP. The machine treats the symptom, not the cause of the problem: obesity. However, the proper management of obesity reverses the condition of chronic obstructive sleep apnea.

Effect of Obesity on Type II Diabetes

Food provides three sources of energy, protein, carbohydrates and fat. Through our digestive and metabolic process, these macronutrients break down into the form of glucose which circulates in the blood. An increase in blood glucose causes the secretion of a hormone from the pancreas called insulin. Insulin facilitates transport of glucose from the blood into the cells of our body to be used for various functions.

Digestion of a meal also causes secretion of glucagon and glucagon-like hormones that will elevate blood sugar and decrease the effect of insulin. This process is known as "insulin resistance". Glucagon and glucagon-like hormones reduce the effect of insulin and its ability to remove glucose from the blood and carry it into the cells. The balance between insulin and glucagon will control our blood sugar level. Lack of insulin or increase in insulin resistance cause an elevation of the blood sugar and this is known as diabetes. The lack of insulin is known as "type I diabetes", an increased insulin resistance is known as "type II diabetes".

Obesity increases insulin resistance which results in elevated blood sugar and the development of type II diabetes. The lack of glucose in our cells causes hunger and food craving (especially for sweets), this vicious circle causes more weight gain and further elevated blood sugar. Diabetes is a debilitating disease. It contributes to three million deaths per year worldwide. Type II diabetes affects twenty-six million Americans, it is estimated that seventy-nine million are pre-diabetic and another seven million who do not even realize that they are diabetic. Consistent high levels of sugar in the blood damages the wall of the blood vessels and leads to hardening of the arteries known as atherosclerosis. Atherosclerosis in coronary arteries can cause premature heart attacks and strokes due to the damage done to the arteries in the heart and brain.

The peripheral vascular disease caused by diabetes, particularly affects the small blood vessels, especially in the lower extremities. It leads to poor circulation and complete blockage or occlusion of the vessels, causing diabetic foot ulcers that easily become infected and can become gangrenous, which results in the amputation and the loss of a limb. The persistent high blood sugar also damages the nerves in the lower extremities. This condition is known as "peripheral neuropathy". Diabetic neuropathy causes the feet become numb and lose protective sensation. This results in unrecognized trauma to the feet. These unrecognized skin injuries easily become infected by the time it is apparent to the individual and will require specialized wound care.

Diabetes is the most common cause of chronic kidney disease, end stage kidney failure and dialysis. This is due to damage to kidney's blood vessels and circulation. This is a progressive condition that eventually results in kidney failure requiring dialysis whereby a machine flushes out the toxins from the blood several times a week.

We see an increased rate of obesity in children and adolescents with the corresponding development of adult type II diabetes mellitus in them. This is quite alarming. The elevated blood sugar levels in children and adolescence greatly affect normal childhood growth. Due to the prevalence of childhood obesity and type II diabetes estimates suggests that for the first time a decrease in the longevity of future generations will be seen.

The process of obesity and type II diabetes is a genetic predisposition with a dominant gene; thus, the incidence of obesity and related type II diabetes increases in each consecutive generation. By the year 2030, current estimates are that close to 90 percent of the population in the United States will be overweight or obese.

It is important to realize type II diabetes in obese individuals is associated with high levels of circulating insulin with increased insulin resistance. Therefore, the treatment of diabetes in these individuals needs to be focused on decreasing insulin resistance and not adding more insulin. If you are diabetic and overweight or obese and have been given insulin to control your blood sugar, you should ask your healthcare provider, "Why are you giving me more insulin? I already have a high level of insulin." Prescribing insulin for obese diabetic people will result in rapid weight gain, which compounds the issue by further increasing insulin resistance which then increases blood glucose levels. This is the exact opposite of the intended effect. Nowadays, in addition to low carbohydrate diets and increased physical activity, we have several new anti-diabetic medications available. These medications primarily will reduce insulin resistance and should be considered as a first line of treatment for obesity related type II diabetes instead of giving more insulin.

When we ingest food, blood sugar increases and as a result insulin is secreted. When food enters the first part of the small intestine called the duodenum it stimulates secretion of a group of glucagon-like hormones resulting in elevated blood sugar and increased insulin resistance. By excluding and bypassing passage of food from the duodenum, we can eliminate the secretion of glucagon-like hormones all together. Such bypass eliminates insulin resistance and circulating insulin will normalize blood sugar in type II diabetes. This surgical procedure is called Roux-en-Y Gastric Bypass (RYGB). It not only normalizes the effects of blood sugar; it also produces an effective weight loss.

The effect of weight loss with RYGB is due to two factors, one is the physical limitation of the size of the stomach and the second is the hormone alteration of the gastrointestinal tract and reduction of insulin resistance. For this reason, after RYGB ingestion of sweets or short chain carbohydrates have uninhibited effects of circulating insulin that will significantly lower blood sugar and causes symptom known as dumping syndrome. It is noted that hormonal changes due to RYGB through a complex repair mechanism that is related to genetic disposition about a few years after RYGB will adapt and glucagon-like hormones will start secreting from other sites in the gastrointestinal tract and eventually their level will rise to pre-surgical level.

This repair mechanism of gastrointestinal hormone is responsible for increased appetite, persistent feeling of hunger and some weight gain a few years after surgery. For a long time, we as surgeons thought that the gastric pouch became enlarged and that was the primary reason for weight gain after surgery. We became more inclined to do Revision of RYGB. However, experience showed that five-year success rate of revisions for additional weight loss is very low. Most of the weight loss effect of RYGB is primarily due to hormonal alteration of the gastrointestinal tract and not the size of the gastric pouch. Reducing the size of gastric pouch has limited effect on weight loss. Weight loss surgery like sleeve gastrectomy does not directly alter insulin resistance, but reducing the size of the stomach and reduced secretion of Ghrelin after sleeve gastrectomy due to weight loss still have favorable results for controlling obesity-related type II diabetes.

Effect of Obesity on the Liver

The liver is the largest internal organ in our body that has multiple functions. It stores a large amount of energy and glucose in the form of glycogen that can be used as a source of energy during fasting and between the meals. Liver also stores iron, vitamins and minerals, it processes proteins and blood clotting factors. Liver also provides bile that helps digest food and fat in the small bowel.

Almost all medications and alcohol will be processed in the liver. It also filters the bacteria that enter our body through the gastrointestinal tract. Liver cells have a remarkable ability to regenerate itself. Obesity will cause fat buildup in the liver cells that will interfere with its healthy function causing scarring of the liver which is known as cirrhosis of the liver. Cirrhosis of the liver is a serious condition and, in some cases, can lead to liver cancer known as hepatocellular carcinoma.

Normally, fat makes up 5-10 percent of the liver. In obesity, the fat percentage of liver is increased and results in a condition known as "steatohepatitis" or fatty infiltration of the liver. This condition will cause altered liver function, enlargement of the liver, elevated liver enzymes and permanent liver damage. Fatty infiltration of the liver in some cases leads to cirrhosis of the liver and liver failure, even cancer of the liver. The global prevalence of childhood obesity is also associated with fatty infiltration of the liver in children and young adults, this situation has shown an increased risk of hepato-cellular carcinoma, which is a type of liver cancer later in adulthood.

It is speculated that changes in the microbial population of the gastrointestinal tract in the obese individual are the cause of absorption of fatty acid and fatty infiltration in the liver cells. Liver biopsies done in the adolescent undergoing weight loss surgery have shown that 60 percent of individuals had fatty liver. Weight loss surgery will improve and reverse fatty infiltration of the liver. In adolescents with obesity and fatty infiltration of the liver should be a strong consideration for weight loss surgery.

It is estimated that 20 percent of the adult population in America suffer from some form of fatty infiltration of the liver. This disease is associated with elevated blood cholesterol, triglycerides, increased insulin resistance and type II diabetes.

Obesity is also associated with gallbladder distention and formation of gallstones.

Weight loss surgery can reverse this condition and improve liver function.

Effect of Obesity on Metabolic Syndrome

The combination of high blood pressure, elevated blood sugar and dyslipidemia (elevated triglycerides and cholesterol) as a result of obesity is called metabolic syndrome. This syndrome is known to worsen the risk of cardiovascular disease such as heart attack and stroke. The most effective treatment of metabolic syndrome is weight loss. Weight loss improves this condition and reduces blood sugar levels, lowers blood pressure as well as triglyceride and cholesterol levels in blood.

Obesity is the most common cause of dyslipidemia, which is defined by elevated low-density lipoprotein (LDL) and cholesterol. Dyslipidemia is an important factor in the development of atherosclerosis that affects coronary arteries and cerebrovascular system and is the leading cause of heart attacks, strokes and premature dcath.

Effect of Obesity on Genitourinary and Reproductive System

Obesity causes urinary disorders in men and women. Overactive bladder, urinary frequency as well as urinary tract infection are more common in obese individuals.

Urinary stress incontinence, particularly in women is associated with obesity. This condition presents itself with loss of bladder control when coughing, sneezing and straining. This condition not only causes social embarrassment, but it interferes with personal hygiene and affects personal activity. This condition improves with weight loss.

Obesity causes sexual dysfunction in both men and women. This affects fertility in both men and women. Obesity causes low testosterone level in men and menstrual disorder in women. Obese women also have a higher risk of miscarriage.

Obesity in women of reproductive age causes development of polycystic ovarian syndrome (PCOS). As obesity is associated with excess levels of insulin with increased insulin resistance, this will affect ovaries to produce excess androgen (male hormone) resulting in ovaries to become enlarged and contain multiple cysts. High androgen levels cause acne and excess facial hair growth. PCOS causes menstrual irregularity and contributes to infertility. Effective weight management will improve PCOS and increase chances of successful pregnancy.

Obesity also increases the risk of several genitourinary cancers in both men and women.

Weight loss surgery has a positive impact on many of these conditions. After weight loss surgery, we witness resolution of many of these conditions.

Effect of Obesity on Musculoskeletal system

Obesity is the most common cause of Gout and inflammatory joint disease. Obesity is also associated with premature degenerative joint disease.

Increased body fat acts as an endocrine organ that produce multiple inflammatory molecules that affect and interact with hormones such as corticosteroids and release multiple by-products that cause tissue aging and inflammatory process in the joints.

Osteoarthritis is a degenerative joint disease that causes substantial disability due to significant joint pain resulting in decreased mobility. Obese individuals are four times more likely to develop osteoarthritis. Osteoarthritis used to be an age-related illness. Obesity is one of the most significant risk factors for the development of early osteoarthritis. Sixty-nine percent of people with this condition are overweight or obese. Osteoarthritis affects cartilage and bone, resulting in premature joint deterioration. This condition is not only caused by the excess weight on weight bearing joints that accelerates the deterioration of the joints, most often osteoarthritis is due to the inflammatory by-products of obesity that affects non-weight bearing joints as well, leading to polyarthritis which is substantially a disabling condition.

Alarmingly, we now see osteoarthritis in children and young adults caused by obesity. This profoundly affects normal children's growth.

Osteoarthritis in obese individuals substantially decrease functional capacity and mobility that contributes to further weight gain.

Treatment of obesity, especially weight loss surgery seems to be the best option of treatment of degenerative joint disorder and obesity related osteoarthritis.

Effect of Obesity on Nervous System: Pseudo-tumor Cerebri

Obesity is a major contributing cause of migraine headaches. In addition, obesity is the cause of severe headaches called pseudo-tumor cerebri.

The brain and spinal cord are surrounded by cerebrospinal fluid. This fluid acts as a cushion to protect the brain and the spinal cord. Increased pressure in the cerebrospinal fluid causes symptoms like having a brain tumor and this condition is called "pseudo-tumor cerebri". Obesity is the main cause of development of this condition. Pseudo-tumor cerebri is twenty times more common in women than men. This condition presents itself with nausea, ringing in the ears and neck and shoulder pain. It also causes headaches that starts behind the eyes and worsens with eye movement. This condition leads to the swelling of the optic nerve and eye vessels that will result in loss of vision and it eventually leads to blindness.

Also, obesity is the major contributory cause of peripheral neuropathy, especially in lower extremities.

Weight loss surgery is the most effective treatment of these conditions.

Effect of Obesity on Development of Cancer

Substantial amounts of research have shown that obesity is associated with the increased risk of development of multiple forms of cancer in men and women. The highest degree of obesity is associated with higher risk of development of cancer.

The hormonal effect and inflammatory process of fatty tissue, promote the biological regulatory system to alter cells into the development of cancer.

In addition, obesity contributes to poor response to cancer treatment and carries a higher risk of surgical complication.

Pancreatic and kidney cancer

Studies show that there is an increased risk of pancreatic and kidney cancer due to obesity in both men and women.

Breast cancer

Obesity is shown to be associated with high levels of estrogen and an increased risk of development of breast cancer in women. Overweight or obese post-menopausal women carry substantially higher risk of developing breast cancer in comparison with normal weight women. In addition, obesity results in poor response to treatment of breast cancer and a high recurrence rate. Progress of breast cancer in both pre and post-menopausal women that are overweight or obese is substantially worse than normal weight women.

Uterine Cancer

Obesity by increasing the estrogen level increases the risk of estrogen-dependent endometrial cancer especially in African American women. The effective treatment of uterine cancer includes hysterectomy. Obesity increases the risks of surgery and its complications such as wound infection, deep vein thrombosis (DVT) and pulmonary embolism (PE). Overall, treatment of uterine cancer in obese women has poor results. Studies show that weight loss surgery is associated with a 71 percent reduction of chance of development of uterine malignancy. In addition, being overweight and obese increases the risk of developing cervical cancer by two folds. Obesity is associated with increased risk of ovarian cancer as well.

Colon Cancer

Obesity has shown to be associated with increased risk of development of colon cancer in men. Such effect is not seen in women. Surgical treatment of colon cancer in obese individuals carries a higher risk of wound infection, non-healing surgical wound and it is associated with higher incidences of DVT and PE. Additionally, obesity is associated with poor response to chemotherapy and poor outcome in comparison with non-obese individuals.

Higher body weight is associated with greater incidences of testicular tumor and more aggressive prostate cancer.

Studies show that weight loss will substantially decrease the risk of development of such cancers.

Effect of Obesity on Skin and Lymphatic System

Obesity is responsible for a variety of skin disorders. Skin functions as a barrier to protect our internal organs from environmental factors and bacteria. Skin also regulates our body temperature. Many dermatological disorders are aggravated by obesity. Obesity causes poor circulation to the skin and results in changes like hyperpigmentation of skin and many others. Friction between skin folds causes skin maceration and accumulation of moisture between the folds that is associated with inadequate hygiene and causes staph and fungal infections of skin. Cellulitis is frequent in obesity that may result in severe systemic infection and require intravenous antibiotic therapy. Some forms of skin infection are called "hidradenitis suppurativa" that results in chronic abscess and skin fistula. Obesity is a common cause of pressure sores and prolonged wound healing.

Excess fatty tissue contributes to increased levels of cortisone, which causes development of stretch marks. These are several bands of skin atrophy with the multiple parallel lines that appear in the abdomen and upper trunk and thighs. This is similar to the stretch marks during pregnancy. With the increase of childhood obesity, we now see the development of stretch marks in children and adolescents. Nowadays 40 percent of obese children in America have stretch marks which are permanent.

Obesity is a common cause of the development of acne and especially facial hair growth in females.

In severe obesity, excess fat distribution in the lower extremities and abdominal area can result in lymphatic blockage and the development of obesity related lymphedema. This condition is known as "lipo-lymphedema", which causes increased fluid in fatty tissue and provides a desirable media for overgrowth of bacteria and fungus and development of cellulitis.

In severe obesity the coping mechanism of storing large amounts of fatty tissue results in the development of large masses that become redundant and heavy due to the effect of gravity and blockage of lymphatic channels causing edema (swelling). These are called lipo-lymphedema masses. These masses become a source of decreased functional ability and are prone to frequent infections. These masses are the result of the ability of the body to store excess fatty tissue. While removal of these masses becomes tempting, however invariably after removal of these masses they will rapidly grow back. Removal of the lipo-lymphedema mass is only indicated after effective weight loss treatment or otherwise will be futile.

After weight loss surgery, redundant excess skin will remain a source of functional disability, repeated infections and the source of dissatisfaction of body image. Skin reduction surgery after significant weight loss improves all undesirable sequela of excess skin.

Effect of Obesity on Gastrointestinal and Digestive System

Excess body weight is associated with abdominal obesity and increases intra-abdominal pressure. This causes a variety of gastrointestinal complaints such as heartburn, abdominal bloating, irritable bowel syndrome (IBS) and bowel irregularity.

Obesity is associated with high incidence of gallbladder disease and formation of gallstones especially in women.

Presence of hiatal hernia and gastroesophageal reflux disease is more common in the obese individuals.

The esophagus is part of the digestive system that connects the mouth to stomach. Esophagus passes through a small opening in the diaphragm which is called the hiatus. Increased intra-abdominal pressure in obese individuals will result in enlargement of diaphragmatic hiatus and protrusion of the stomach into the hiatus and above the diaphragm. This is called "hiatal hernia". This condition is associated with the frequent gastro-esophageal reflux of food and acid into the lower segment of esophagus. This results in chronic inflammation of the esophagus that is known as "esophagitis". Esophagitis presents with heartburn and chest pain. Gastroesophageal reflux disease worsens by lying down, especially at night and it can become a source of aspiration of food into the trachea and respiratory system and even affecting the vocal cords.

Hiatal hernia and chronic aspiration can be a cause of chronic bronchitis, pneumonia and even lung abscess.

Chronic gastroesophageal reflux disease may lead to a condition called Barrett's esophagus. This condition is precancerous and if left untreated will result in cancer of the esophagus.

Hiatal hernia can be treated with anti-reflux medication, but in severe cases may require surgical repair. It should be noted that surgical repair of hiatal hernia alone without treatment of obesity, carry a high incidence of failure. An effective management of obesity and weight loss surgery will dramatically improve gastrointestinal disorders associated with obesity.

Psychological Effect of Obesity

Obesity and related illnesses are predisposing factors for the development of mood alteration and emotional difficulties. Obese individuals are at greater risk of developing depression and anxiety. In some cases, depression may be the underlying cause of obesity. It seems there is a positive correlation between obesity and depression. This is considered the bidirectional risk between the development of depression and obesity. It is unknown which condition existed first, did the depression cause the obesity or did the obesity cause the depression?

Studies have shown that these depressive emotional difficulties and mood alterations are more prevalent in obese individuals. Obesity will negatively impact the overall quality of life and an individual's self-esteem. Additionally, society's attitude towards obesity and biased opinion with discriminatory attitude will promote isolation and loss of social ability in many obese individuals. Invariably obese individuals become more homebound and find comfort by utilizing food which results in more weight gain.

The psychological effect of obesity as well as the lack of physical activity promotes the tendency for seeking a codependent symbiotic relationship to find comfort with food. Usually an enabler who approves of and endorses this faulty eating habits and self-destructive behavior will exert their control over the obese individual by fulfilling their role in providing the food to show that they are needed and love the obese individual.

Breaking free from the enabler can be extremely difficult. The emotional abuse in fear of disappointment in the physical and emotional dependency upon the enabler by the obese individual is difficult to overcome. This codependency on the enabler maybe one of the most difficult challenges in the aspect of the treatment of obesity, since the obese person will continue their faulty eating habits due to the fear of loss of the symbiotic relationship with the enabler.

One of the most dramatic psychological effects on the obese individual with poor health is the daily suffering due to the diminish quality of life. This results in a sense of hopelessness that increases the risk of suicide in many obese individuals.

The psychological effect of social bias, discrimination and bullying significantly increase risk of suicide especially in the youth population. This should not be taken lightly because suicide is the third cause of death among the youth population particularly in young girls. Complexity of psychological issues in obese individuals along with their addictive personalities shouldn't be overlooked in misusage of drugs, alcohol and tobacco.

It is clear that weight loss surgery will have a positive impact in the return of self-esteem and the ability to increase social skills and therefore it reduces anxiety and depression.

* * *

Chapter 7
Digestive and metabolic process, dietary balance and regulation of feeding

Food plays a significant role in our life and it is essential for our survival. Hunger, the desire for food intake, the feeling of satiety as well as energy expenditure in our body are regulated by a complex metabolic process. This process which regulates our food intake and energy expenditure will affect our weight. If the food intake exceeds the energy expenditure it results in weight gain. The energy provided from food is expressed by **calories**. The process by which food is broken down in our body to provide nutrients and energy is called **digestive process**. The process by which our body converts nutrients to energy is called the **metabolic process**.

Digestive Process

The digestive process is a process that converts food into smaller particles that can be easily absorbed from our digestive system into our body so that it can provide the required energy for our daily functions. Digestive process consists of two separate functions.

One is a **mechanical function** that consists of food intake with our mouth and the passage of food into our digestive system and provides waste product for elimination. This process is by mechanical passage of food throughout the digestive system with muscular contractions of our digestive system that is called peristalsis.

The other function of digestive system is a **chemical process**, by using digestive enzymes and gastric acid and chemical function of gastrointestinal microbiota, the food is broken down into small particles that can be easily absorbed from our intestinal tract into our body for immediate use of energy and bodily function. Each area of the digestive system provides specific mechanical and chemical function.

Our gastrointestinal tract hosts several microorganisms that are referred to as gastrointestinal microflora. These microorganisms are essential for the function of the gastrointestinal system and metabolic process. It is estimated that approximately 30 trillion microorganisms reside in our gastrointestinal tract. That accounts for a total of 2 to 5 pounds of weight in an adult person. Gut microbiota has a symbiotic relationship with our body and provide us with a healthy digestive process as well as metabolic process. These bacteria influence gastrointestinal epithelium for motility and extraction of calories from the food. Microbial colonization of human gastrointestinal tract starts at birth. Babies' microflora is similar to their mothers. In addition to establishing healthy function of our gastrointestinal tract they also support our immune system and protect our gastrointestinal system against harmful bacteria. New emerging clarity indicates that our metabolism is highly influenced by our gastrointestinal microflora and recent shift in our gut microbiota can explain developmental metabolic disorders such as obesity, type II diabetes and cardiovascular disease.

The digestive process begins with the mouth, by chewing the food and swallowing. After food is swallowed it moves down the esophagus. The esophagus is a muscular tube which carries food from the mouth to the stomach. The stomach can hold a sizable amount of food usually about three pints. The stomach then releases the food in small increments through its outlet that is called pylorus. The food released from the stomach moves into the first portion of the intestine which is called duodenum. Then the food moves further down into the small intestine for absorption. The small intestine is about 20 to 30 feet long and provide for absorption of nutrients from the food. The upper part of the intestine is called jejunum, and the lower part is called ileum. The remaining food then moves into the large intestine which is called colon. The water is absorbed through the colon and waste products are stored in for elimination.

The chemical function of the digestive enzymes with acid of our gastrointestinal microbiota starts in the mouth with salivary enzymes that start the breakdown of the food. This process continues in the stomach, gastric juices and enzymes breakdown the food to smaller particles. In the duodenum bile and pancreatic enzymes further break down the food, especially proteins and fat and other nutrients. There will be further digestive enzymes and microbial function in the small bowel to provide further breakdown of food to finer elements that will be absorbed in the small bowel into our blood flow and body. The nutrients that are absorbed in our body will be converted to energy by the metabolic process.

Our digestive system can store a sizable amount of food that can provide us with source of energy for many hours. Normally it takes 6 to 8 hours for a digestive process to be completed. Therefore, it is not necessary for us to eat more frequently than 2 or 3 times a day. Contrary to a common myth, eating frequently does not simulate or speed up our metabolism.

* * *

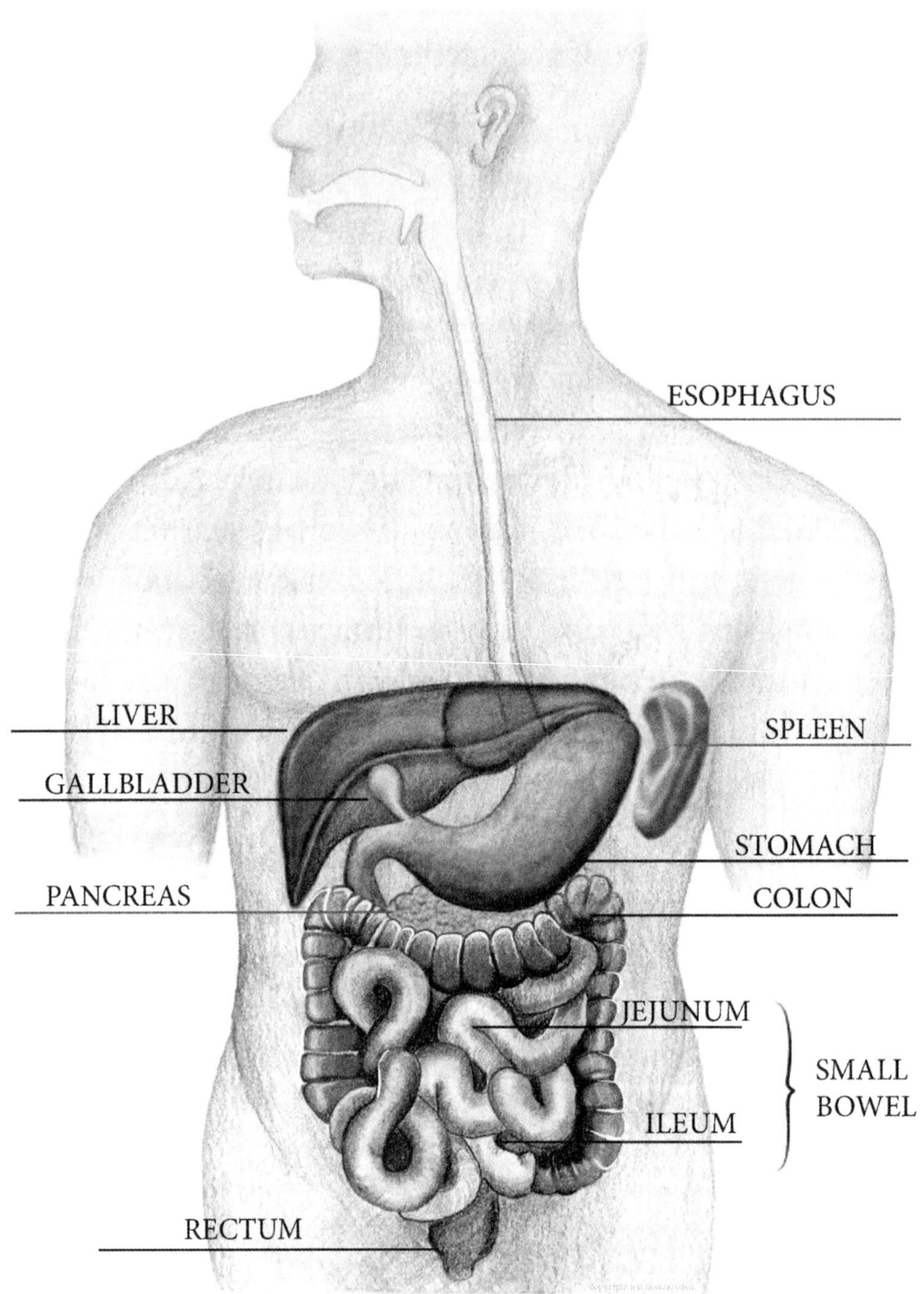

DIGESTIVE SYSTEM

Metabolic process

Complex physiological factors and metabolic processes that create desire for food intake and satiety feeling that inhibits food intake is regulated in the central brain in the hypothalamus. Multiple chemicals and neurohormonal signals pathway convey messages to hypothalamus which regulates our food intake and energy expenditure. Multiple hormones released from the stomach and gastrointestinal tract and many peripheral hormones as well as adipose tissue, affect the neurohormonal pathway. In addition, the chemical signals such as level of blood glucose and fatty acid and amino acid will have additional input. Also signals from cerebral cortex such as sense of smell or taste or vision of food will have effect on our regulatory center in hypothalamus. These regulatory mechanisms not only affect our food intake but also affect our energy expenditure.

The gastrointestinal microbiota also plays a key role in our metabolic process. Certain gastrointestinal microbes influence the gut epithelium and its mobility to extract more calories from the food. Our gut microbiota acts as if it is a separate endocrine organ that contribute to desensitization of insulin signaling pathway that influences our food intake and calories storage and it plays a key role in developing obesity, type II diabetes and cardiovascular disease.

There are three sources of energy in our food, **carbohydrates**, **protein** and **fat**. They are all absorbed in our body in the form of glucose, which is a form of an ordinary sugar. The energy absorbed from the food intake will be used for immediate daily bodily functions.

An average person utilizes between 50 to 80 calories per hour. Physical activities can increase body's calorie consumption. The reminder of the energy that is being provided by the food will be converted to glucagon which is a polysaccharide. Glucagon will be stored in our body for future use between the meals as a source of energy. Glucagon is stored in the liver and muscles. Liver can store a generous amount of energy that can be used for many hours and sometimes days. If the energy intake from the food exceeds the amount that is being used or stored in the liver and muscle, then it will be stored in the form of fat in our body for future use as a source of energy.

Due to ability of liver to store generous amount of energy that can be used between meals, we do not need to eat frequently. Three or even two meals a day provide more than enough source or energy for our body.

The complex process of regulatory mechanism which affects the food intake in our body includes several hormones, the nervous system and the hypothalamus in the brain. During fasting a polypeptide hormone called Ghrelin is secreted from the stomach. This hormone stimulates the neuropathways to the hypothalamus in the brain and creates the feeling of appetite, hunger and the desire to eat. Additionally, visual stimulation of food or sensory stimulation of smell can trigger the neurohormonal pathways to the hypothalamus can create the desire for food. Eating and presence of food in the stomach and gastric distention will signal suppression of Ghrelin and our hunger will subside, however, this process may take a while to develop. If we eat too fast, we may get physically full before our desire for food completely subside which invariably results in overeating. Not eating for long periods of time may result in a profound sense of hunger that takes much longer after eating to dissipate and usually results in over eating.

Passage of the food through the intestinal system also stimulates production of multiple pancreatic and intestinal hormones that through the neurohormonal pathway will further inhibit our food intake and eliminate the desire to eat. For this reason, many individuals who do not eat all day and overeat late at night, the next morning have no desire to eat. They will invariably skip breakfast and will not get hungry until later in the day. This habit is known as the night eating syndrome. Night eating syndrome is always associated with obesity due to over eating. Another form of an eating disorder is binge eating which always results in obesity; frequent eating in small amount always results in excessive intake of calories and loss of control of eating.

Our central digestion neurohormonal pathway to hypothalamus is also affected by many peripheral hormones. These hormones are secreted from other organs such as the thyroid, adrenal, ovaries, testicle and fat cells in our body. These hormones are growth hormone thyroxin, corticosteroid, insulin, progesterone, testosterone, estrogen, leptin and many others. These hormones not only regulate our calorie intake but also effect energy output and calorie expenditure as well.

The key role that gastrointestinal microbiome play in our metabolism is becoming clearer to be responsible for calorie intake and calorie expenditure. The changes in our gastrointestinal microbiota are known as dysbiosis. This shift in our gastrointestinal tract microbiota plays a significant role in metabolic segments that are causing increased calorie absorption from the food and increased appetite and fat storage. Although quite complex, there is clearly an association with development of obesity and metabolic disorder such as type II diabetes, and cardiovascular disease. The gut microbiota act as a separate endocrine organ that affects our metabolic process and influences desensitization of insulin signaling pathways which increase the risk of diabetes.

Ideally the metabolic process of daily energy intake from food and daily energy expenditure are balanced so our body weight will remain stable. When the calorie intake from food exceeds the energy expenditure by the body, the excess energy will be stored in our body in the form of fat. Over time this will result in weight gain and obesity. When the calorie intake from food is decreased energy expenditure still exist and will require calories to meet the energy expenditure. Therefore, we will use stored energy in the form of fat in our body; as a result, we lose weight. This condition is best seen in anorexia, lack of appetite and after weight loss surgery.

Due to the ability of the stomach to hold large quantities of food, and it takes six to eight hours to complete the digestive process after each meal along with the ability of the liver to store a considerable amount of energy, it is not necessary to eat frequently. Eating three times or even two times a day is enough to provide our daily energy requirements. Eating more than two or three times a day contrary to popular myth does not alter or speed up our metabolism and is not compatible with our normal digestive system function. In addition, frequent eating and grazing results in loss of control for eating.

The complex metabolic process that controls our food intake can be significantly influenced by environmental factors that control our eating habits. These eating habits usually have developed over years and can override the efficiency of the metabolic process and result in obesity. It is best to eat two or three times a day. We should chew our food thoroughly and take time to eat in order to allow time for satiety to develop and the sensation of fullness. We should take at least 20 minutes for each meal to eat. Currently, fast food drive through service have become the life style choice to accommodate a modern busy life. Many of us eat fast and eat in the car; this always results in over eating high calorie foods.

We should not go hungry for a long period of time since it takes much longer after we eat for the sense of hunger to dissipate and always results in over eating.

Many changes have occurred in the modern food environment that promote overconsumption of food. Global and personal economic growth with changes in our food supply that is inexpensive is an important factor. There is a rapid growth of worldwide supermarkets and fast food restaurants that provide inexpensive food which is widely and readily available. Food industry in a competitive market has chemically altered and highly processed the food for rapid digestion and frequent food consumption. They produce calorie concentrated foods which are high in sugar and fat content and chemically altered to develop an addictive taste. They also use marketing strategies such as supersized portions of food or sugary drinks and as result create a permissive environment for overconsumption of food that has become a worldwide phenomenon.

Our metabolism is the result of many genes that regulate the interaction of multiple hormones of the central digestive system, peripheral hormone that regulate food intake and calorie expenditure that as a result dictate our weight. The hormonal-make up and genetic predispositions that controls calorie intake and calorie expenditure varies from person to person. Daily calorie requirement of each person is different.

Control of appetite and predisposition of obesity have been linked to 41 sites on the human genoma. Genetic predisposition of obesity is in our DNA. A single genetic defect causing obesity (monogenetic) is a rare condition. In this case child exhibits an excessive desire for food since birth and child exhibits obesity early in life. Any obesity prior to age 5 should be evaluated for genetic testing. This single gene cause of obesity known as monogenetic for obesity is rare. One form of monogenetic is known as Congenital Leptin Deficiency.

Leptin is a hormone that is secreted from adipocytes (fat cells) which inhibit the effect of Ghrelin in hypothalamus and also acts on peripheral organs and improves insulin sensitivity. Ghrelin is a hormone that is secreted from the stomach during fasting that creates feeling of hunger and desire to eat. Treating leptin deficiency with leptin, leads to a remarkable reversal of obesity.

Other monogenetic cause of obesity which are rare known as POMC deficiency, Bardet-Biedl syndrome and Prader-Willi syndrome. These are defects in neurohormonal pathway to hypothalamus that cause early childhood obesity.

More often genetic predisposition of obesity is a result of several genes that control multiple hormones. This genetic predisposition of obesity cannot be altered by dietary changes and exercise. In many cases it is not a person's choice and it is not entirely due to lack of discipline and will power, it is simply outside of a person's control. The genetic predisposition of severe obesity cannot be altered with diet and exercise. Weight loss surgery has been proven to be the most effective option for correcting the metabolic process of obesity. Weight loss surgery aside from limiting the amount of food intake also alters the neurohormonal response to a more appropriate level. These hormonal changes after weight loss surgery seem to play a more important role in weight loss than the limiting factor.

Aside from these genes that are in our DNA, there are many inheritable genes that are not in our DNA. These genes remain dormant in our body. Biological regulatory system throughout our body is responsive to the environmental factors which modify hereditary gene expression without altering DNA sequence. These dormant genes can be turned on and become active. This is called epigenetic modification that can also play a role in hereditary causes of obesity.

Obesity is a complex metabolic condition that is multifactorial and multidimensional. The simplified frame work of metabolism and energy expenditure that was mentioned earlier in this chapter can be also highly influenced by multiple other complex processes in many other dimensions. These various complex matters that effect obesity are partly related to environmental factors such as family and household dynamics and presence of an enabler, psychological factors such as depression and many others. The complex contributing factors in the development of obesity varies from person to person. Therefore, the potential for obesity is different in each individual.

The treatment objectives for obesity should be focused on identifying and addressing all contributory factors involved. In dealing with obesity we should consider the person as a whole and complex circumstance surrounding their lives, including their intellectual and educational level. We need to understand their emotional and psychological issues. We should also consider their cultural background, household dynamics and interrelationship with others. A single solution is not going to fit everyone. If a hammer is the only tool we have, then everything else is going to look like a nail. A cookie cutter treatment of obesity in many cases has a short-term success, often we see weight gain resurface after someone has had weight loss surgery. In most cases, the causes of contributory factors leading to obesity were not adequately addressed. Such treatment in the long run results in disappointment as well as frustration of repeated unsuccessful weight loss. There is an abundance of different modalities of weight loss diets, medications, and remedies. These various options of treatment contribute to an array of many contradictory and confusing options for treatment that not only results in failure of treatment but the development of a faulty foundation and many erroneous opinions regarding this matter. Building on a faulty foundation inevitably collapses on itself. Since we cannot know what we don't know, knowledge is going to be the key factor to success. Therefore, we should keep an open mind and forget what we think we know and build a foundation based on proven scientific facts.

Our role as physicians is to identify all contributory factors involved in development of obesity and develop a plan which addresses all the issues to ensure long-term success. Looking for solutions without knowing what the problem is will never succeed. It almost seems as if we need to go somewhere, but we don't know where we are going so, we will never get there.

* * *

Chapter 8
Childhood and adolescent obesity

Obesity has become a modern day worldwide epidemic and it is one of the most challenging public health problems of our time. Currently, obesity is affecting nearly one out of three adults in the world. Since 1980, obesity has doubled in 70 countries in the world. In 2015 four million deaths in the world were attributed to obesity. For centuries childhood obesity was a rare occasion. In 1836 Charles Dickens in novel called "The Pickwick papers", describes a fat boy as puffy adolescent who is constantly hungry, very red in the face and always falling asleep. In 1918 William Osler, founder of Johns Hopkins university, describes Pickwickian syndrome that encompassed obesity hypoventilation and somnolence.

In the past few decades childhood and adolescent obesity appeared to be increasing at an alarming rate in the world as well as in the United States. The recent studies show that over 180 million children globally have a BMI of over 30 kg/m^2. Over the past 3 decades in the United States the incidences of childhood obesity have more than tripled and at the same time the incidents of the adolescent obesity have nearly quadrupled. Severe obesity is currently known to be as a fast-growing problem in the youth. Currently, in the United States 32 percent of children between the ages of 10 and 17 are overweight and 17 percent are considered to be obese.

In 2015, the United States had the highest percentage of childhood obesity in the world. In the past 10 years in the United States, military recruits rejected for weight problem has jumped from 12 percent to 21 percent. An overweight adolescent has a 70 percent chance of becoming overweight or obese as an adult; this risk is increased by more than 80 percent if the parents are overweight or obese. Nowadays multi-generation obesity has become a common occurrence in our society. Obese children when compared with non-obese ones face 10 to 20 years decrease in their life expectancy. Many of these youth will develop health conditions in their 20s that are typically seen in 40 to 60 years-old. It is predicted that for the first time that longevity of an entire future generation will decrease due to obesity. It is predicted that in our country, obesity will become not only the leading cause of premature death, but also a leading cause of preventable death. It is also predicted that in the very near future for the first time in the modern times, we will witness a sustained drop in our life expectancy due to today's obesity problems. It is estimated that in the next few decades, life expectancy of an average American will decline by more than five years. Many obese children and adolescents have significant comorbidities that are typically seen in adults such as obstructive sleep apnea, hypertension, enlarged heart, hyperlipidemia, fatty infiltration of liver, gout and depression. Now for the first time we see elevated hemoglobin A1C and adult Type II diabetes in children as a result of obesity.

Obesity also impacts health related quality of life in children and adolescents; joint pain and impaired body composition invariably results in decreased cognitive skills and inability to participate in physical activity and fitness programs. The increase in visceral fat negatively impacts healthy brain function. Obesity stigma and bias in children of school age causes poor social skills and lack of participation, resulting in isolation and depression as well. Depression, bullying and internet use in recent years has led to significant increase in youth suicide particularly in young girls. The psychological impact in youth should not be taken lightly since suicide is the third leading cause of death among young population and represents a significant public health problem worldwide.

Obesity and sedentary life style is one of the most challenging public health problems of our time, and it is affecting nearly one out of three people in the world. In 2015 four million deaths in the world were contributed to obesity.

Obesity related cardiovascular disease in children and adolescent.

Dramatic impact of obesity on cardiovascular disease is one of the causes of premature death. There is paralleled prevalence of increasing risk of cardiovascular disease with any degree of obesity in youth. Obesity will cause an increase in cardiac load and elevated blood pressure and increases vascular resistance. Increased cardiac load and vascular resistance will cause enlargement of heart muscle known as ventricular hypertrophy. Ventricular hypertrophy due to strain in heart muscle causes irregular heartbeat as well as structural changes of heart muscle causing cardiomyopathy. Also we see pulmonary hypertension and risk of adulthood premature death, severe obesity in youth is also associated with other comorbidities like type II diabetes mellitus, and dyslipidemia that will cause elevated inflammatory marker and will increase risk of premature arteriosclerosis or hardening of the arteries in early ages, effect of high blood pressure on kidneys results in chronic kidney disease or early kidney failure.

Cardiovascular disease associated with childhood and adolescent will significantly decrease functional capacity and leads to sedentary lifestyle. Treatment of childhood and adolescent obesity will significantly improve cardiovascular risk factors.

Obesity related respiratory illnesses in children and adolescent.

Many obese children and adolescent suffer from hypoventilation syndrome. The excess weight on the chest and respiratory muscles along with elevated diaphragm due to abdominal obesity restricts lung capacity and its function. Hypoventilation syndrome decreases the ability for activity and exercise and is associated with shortness of breath and rapid heartbeat. Hypoventilation syndrome along with hypertension can result in pulmonary hypertension which is a cause of significant risk of morbidity and mortality in adult life.

Nearly one third of obese children and adolescents suffer from obstructive sleep apnea. Sleep apnea is due to narrowing of upper airway and along with hypoventilation is associated with habitual snoring and low level of oxygen and increased carbon dioxide in the blood, that results in intermittent secession of breading during sleep that forces requiring to wake up to start breading. This condition is associated with poor sleep and causes morning headaches and being drowsy and sleepy during the daytime. Obstructive sleep apnea is caused by difficulty in falling asleep and the daytime difficulty with attention problem and being irritable. This condition is associated with a significant decrease in healthy quality-of-life and increased risk of morbidity and mortality in adolescent. While this condition requires positive pressure devices during the bedtime, it is a strong indication that surgical intervention should be considered when dealing with obstructive sleep apnea in adolescent.

Obesity related Type II diabetes mellitus in children and adolescent.

There is paralleled increase in insulin resistance and Type II diabetes mellitus in obese children and adolescent worldwide. Presence of Type II diabetes mellitus in children and adolescent is a predictor of increased rate of death from cardiovascular disease. Studies show that a decline in insulin secreting cells of the pancreas is 4 times faster than adults and kidney disease occurs earlier in adolescent than adults. In addition, retinopathy (eye disease) and elevated blood sugar damages to peripheral nerves causing neuropathy and neuropsychiatric condition of diabetes are more severe in adolescents than are in adults. Childhood and adolescent Type II diabetes mellitus needs effective interventional therapy.

Obesity related idiopathic intracranial hypertension in children and adolescent.

Idiopathic intracranial hypertension is known as pseudotumor cerebri and is a condition of increased pressure inside the skull in the fluid surrounding the brain. There is a strong association between childhood and adolescent obesity and increased intracranial pressure. This condition has symptoms that mimic a brain tumor such as headache and blurred vision and left untreated can cause blindness. Other symptoms include nausea, vomiting and dizziness ringing in the ears and neck and shoulder pain. This condition can be treated with a shunt from the fluid surrounding brain or spine into the abdominal cavity to decrease pressure inside the skull. In the case of adolescent obesity and pseudotumor cerebri weight loss surgery should be strongly considered.

Obesity related liver dysfunction in children and adolescents.

One of the obesity related conditions in children and adolescents is known as fatty infiltration of the liver. Liver is the largest organ in our body that has multiple functions. It stores a large amount of energy and the glucose in the form of glycogen that can be used as a source of energy during fasting and between meals. Liver also stores iron, vitamins and minerals. It produces proteins and blood clotting factors. Liver also produces bile that helps digest food and fat in the small bowel. Most of medications and alcohol will be processed in the liver. It also filters the bacteria that enter our body through gastrointestinal tract. Liver has a remarkable ability to regenerate itself. Obesity will cause fat buildup in the liver cells that will interfere with healthy function of liver and causing scarring of liver which is known as cirrhosis of the liver. Cirrhosis of the liver is a serious condition and, in some cases, can lead to liver cancer known as hepatocellular carcinoma.

Changes in the microbial population of gastrointestinal tract in the obese individual is the cause of absorption of fatty acid and fatty infiltration in the liver cells. Liver biopsies done in the adolescent undergoing weight loss surgery have shown that 60 percent of individuals had fatty liver. Weight loss surgery will improve and reverse fatty infiltration of the liver. Adolescents with obesity and fatty infiltration liver should be strongly considered for weight loss surgery.

Orthopedic complications of obesity in childhood and adolescent

There are pediatric orthopedic complications of obesity that are not seen in adults. The weight of obesity during growth in children and adolescent has highest impact on growth plate of tibia (shin bone) just below the knees. Failure of development of growth plate will result in angling of the bone that is known as bowed leg known as tibia vara or Blount disease. In many cases this condition requires orthopedic procedures however weight loss surgery must be considered prior to orthopedic procedure.

Another weight related orthopedic complication of childhood and adolescent obesity is slipped capital femoral epiphysis (SCFE). In this condition the ball of the head of the femur (thighbone) slips off the neck of the bone in a backwards direction causing pain and stiffness of hip. This requires orthopedic procedure but weight loss procedure must be done before orthopedic procedure.

Gastrointestinal complication of obesity in children and adolescent.

One of the common complications of pediatric obesity, caused by increased intra-abdominal pressure is gastroesophageal reflux disease and development of sliding type hiatal hernia. This condition is associated with reflux and regurgitation of food or liquids in esophagus, difficulty in swallowing and risk of aspiration in lungs, and can present with symptoms of asthma. Severe gastroesophageal reflux in children and adolescent is a strong consideration for weight loss surgery.

Understanding childhood and adolescent obesity

Childhood obesity is defined as a condition of excess fat accumulation in the body that would adversely affect their well-being. We use body mass index (BMI) to quantify the degree of obesity. A normal BMI is considered to be between 18 to 25 kg/m^2, a BMI of 25 to 30 kg/m^2 is considered being overweight, a BMI of 30 to 40 kg/m^2 is considered to be obese, and a BMI greater than 40 kg/m^2 is known as severe obesity. Considering a BMI variation for age group, gender and ethnic background. BMI calculation is done by multiplying weight in pounds by 703 and dividing height in inches twice. A 150-pound child with a height of 4 feet has a BMI of 45.77 kg/m^2: 150x703 ÷48 ÷48 =45.77

Children as young as two years old should be evaluated and screened for being overweight and obese. Many obese children suffer from many comorbid conditions that are typically seen in adults such as obstructive sleep apnea, hypoventilation syndrome and respiratory difficulties, high blood pressure, enlarged heart with increased cardiac load, type II diabetes, osteoarthritis and depression. Pediatric obesity is based on genetic predisposition and is influenced by permissive environment that start in vitro and extends through childhood and adolescent and threatens their adulthood health and longevity.

Endocrine etiology in childhood obesity is a rare occurrence and usually is associated with other development symptoms. Genetic screening is only indicated in early childhood obesity before age 5, this rare condition is usually due to a single gene causing obesity and this is known as Congenital Leptin Deficiency. Leptin is a hormone that is produced by adipose cells that help regulate energy balance by inhibiting action of a hormone called ghrelin. Ghrelin is a hormone that causes hunger. Both hormones act on hypothalamus which is the area of the brain that controls appetite and energy consumption. Congenital lack of leptin by absence of suppression of ghrelin will result in excessive hunger and congenital obesity. In the case of congenital obesity, children from birth experience an excessive appetite and become obese soon after birth. Other single gene (monogenetic) causes of obesity are known as POMC deficiency syndrome and Prader-Willi syndrome.

However, the genetic predisposition of obesity more often is due to the interaction of multiple genes that regulates numerous hormones that effect food intake and cellular energy consumption. These hormones are growth hormones, insulin, thyroxine, corticosteroids, estrogen, progesterone, testosterone, glucagon, ghrelin and various gastrointestinal hormones that affect insulin resistance and food metabolism. Aside from the DNA genes, there are many inheritable genes that are not in our DNA. These genes remain dormant in our body. Biological regulatory systems which are present throughout our body, in response to the environmental factors can modify these hereditary gene expressions without altering our DNA sequence. This response is called an epigenetic modification. This results in the transmission of emotional and behavioral pattern from the parents to the child which results in a similar pattern of eating disorders in children.

Children ages 6 and older should be screened for obesity and intensive treatment featuring exercise and nutritional counseling should be implemented also. Intervention in childhood and adolescent obesity requires changes in the dynamics of the entire family and the household that focuses on healthy eating habits and changes from sedentary lifestyle to an active one.

Childhood and adolescent obesity is a worldwide growing problem. Dealing with childhood and adolescent obesity is more complex than dealing with adult obesity. We are dealing with a child that we have to consider their level of maturity, intelligence and education to comprehend the scope of the problem and magnitude of treatment. We are also dealing with the parents and the entire household dynamic as well as social, cultural and emotional issues and dietary habits that involve the entire family. We must not forget the child interaction with peers in school and the emotional factors involved. We should consider as a factor the parents state of obesity and the struggle they have with their eating habits. We should make sure that there will be no disagreement between parent and child regarding the plan of treatment.

Considering the complexity of the matter, a coordinated team approach that includes social worker, dietitian, therapist and pediatrician or primary care physician is necessary to ensure successful and durable outcome of treatment. Children of ages 10 to 19 that have a BMI greater than 35 kg/m^2 should be considered for treatment. The first step in the treatment plan should include lifestyle change involving not only the child but the entire family and household. Appropriate dietary changes along with the implementation of physical activity must be initiated. Invariably a social worker would be helpful to address household dynamical and economics, and a dietitian to initiate healthy eating habits.

Any emotional issue such as parents and family dispute, physical and sexual abuse, needs to be properly addressed with a therapist. Neither of these conditions are contraindication for surgical treatment. Status of bone growth also is not a factor for consideration of weight loss surgery. In the meantime, appropriate obesity medication can be implemented to achieve the best results. In case of severe obesity with a BMI greater than 40 kg/m^2 and comorbid conditions, surgical option should be strongly considered.

Considering the child's level of maturity, the risk and benefit of surgery should be explained to the child as well as both parents or caregivers and there should not be any disagreement between child and the parents regarding the plan of treatment and choice of surgical procedure. They should be informed regarding the lifelong commitment of use of vitamin and supplements and lifelong follow-up. Pediatric weight loss program should have transition to adulthood and appropriate follow up. Both parents and child need to understand that failure of the procedure can occur. Pediatric weight loss surgery programs ensure the safety and quality of outcome. The risk of surgery and complications are far less than the risk of obesity and comorbid condition.

Studies suggest that bariatric surgery is more effective than diet and exercise alone for treatment of obesity in children and adolescents. Surgery should be considered for adolescents with BMI greater than forty and BMI greater than thirty-five with serious co-morbid conditions. Despite of safety and effectiveness of adolescent weight loss surgery, there is a large disparity in percentage of weight loss surgery for adults compared to children. Despite studies showing an increase in the prevalence of childhood obesity and related co morbid diseases, the utilization of weight loss surgery in the past few years has not increased.

In the past year approximately one hundred sixty thousand weight loss surgeries were performed on the adults in the United States of which only a thousand of such procedures were performed on the adolescents. This lack of utilization of weight loss surgery in adolescents seems to be multifactorial. What seems to be partially responsible for this underutilization of weight loss surgery for adolescents is the lack of referral by primary care physicians and pediatricians and their hesitance to recommend weight loss surgery. The insurance barrier seems even more challenging for the adolescent than the adult population. Other factors involve concern about psychological issucs involving the care giver and the level of maturity of the adolescent. Finally, the concern about the medical liability issues and extended statute of limitation in children and adolescent has impacted the level of utilization for weight loss surgery.

* * *

Chapter 9
Nutrition

Most diseases are often related to our dietary habits in the first place. So that means that they can be reversed with a proper diet. Some of them are genetic and we may be a carrier of the gene, but it is not guaranteed that it will become active. In this chapter I will give you the details of a few things that we can do to minimize the risk of a genetic condition from becoming active. Our health is our greatest wealth, we must realize that we do have a say in our lives and what our fate is. Our dietary habits dictate our longevity and our behaviors affect our life expectancy. We live the life we choose.

Adequate nutrition is essential for our body to provide energy for our daily metabolic process. The sources of nutrition are divided in two groups. The first group is called macronutrients, such as protein, carbohydrates and fat. Macronutrients are the primary source of our energy. The other group is known as micronutrients which include minerals and vitamins. Micronutrients are an important part of proper nutrition and necessary for our metabolic process. Different foods contain different proportions of proteins, carbohydrates, fats, minerals and vitamins. Appropriate balance with our food intake must be maintained to optimize proper nutrition. Poor dietary selection and habits, coupled with the reduced vitamin and mineral content of food, results in nutritional deficiencies. Being overweight or obese is associated with excessive calorie intake but not necessarily indicative of proper nutritional state. Many obese individuals are undernourished and significantly deficient in micronutrients.

Most often obese individuals suffer from low protein and albumin levels as well as significant vitamins and minerals deficiency. Although their dietary intake consists of excessive calories, it contains low protein, low minerals and vitamins. Dietary protein should be the priority of calorie intake. Low protein intake may lead to low lean body mass instead of low body fat. Nutritional screening and assessment should be considered when dealing with obesity. Most often nutritional intervention by a physician or clinical dietitian is necessary to address malnutrition in obese or overweight individuals. This assessment is particularly important when weight loss surgery is considered. After weight loss surgery nutritional deficiency will be exacerbated due to the altered absorption and limitation on the amount of food intake.

Macronutrients

Macronutrients are the primary source of energy from food. There are three forms of energy source; **carbohydrates, fats and proteins.**

Carbohydrates

Carbohydrates are the most common source of energy. Most foods contain carbohydrates. The energy produces from each gram of carbohydrates produces 4 calories. There are two forms of carbohydrates, simple and complex. Carbohydrates are the most non-essential part of our nutrition. According to the USDA Food Guide released in the early 1990's, daily caloric intake from carbohydrates should be limited and not to exceed 40 percent of one's daily calorie intake.

Simple carbohydrates

Simple carbohydrates are a short chain carbohydrate that are easily digested and rapidly absorbed. They provide an immediate source of energy that usually lasts for short period of time. Simple carbohydrates include sugar, candies, cookies, ice cream and sweet fruits.

Complex carbohydrates

Complex carbohydrates are long chain carbohydrates. Complex carbohydrates take a longer time to digest and absorb. They create a slower and steady source of energy that lasts a longer period of time. Complex carbohydrates include bread, pasta, rice, potato, corn and starches. Most food products contain high amount of carbohydrates. Carbohydrates are the major cause of excess daily calorie intake. Daily calorie intake from carbohydrates is limited as much as possible. In addition, any weight loss diet should be very low in carbohydrates.

Protein

Proteins are the most essential and efficient sources of energy from food. One gram of protein produces 4 calories of energy. Our body does not manufacture protein therefore we require protein in our daily diet. Protein is used in our body for muscles, bones, skin, blood and hormones. Protein is essential for healing, immunity against illnesses, for the structure, function and regulation of all the body's tissues and organs. It performs nearly every function performed by the body at the cellular level. Proteins provide for a slow steady release of energy rather than the ups and downs that we experience with carbs and sugar. A steady diet lacking sufficient amount of protein results in a breakdown of our body's protein. That leads to numerous health issues. Daily calorie intake of protein should be at least 40 percent of the total calorie intake. This is 50 – 120 grams per day depending upon body habits and our activity level. Protein sources include meat, chicken, turkey, seafood, fish and plant-based proteins.

Protein-Rich foods

FOOD ITEM	SERVING SIZE	AMOUNT OF PROTEIN (GRAM)
Beans, baked	½ cup	6
Beans, refried (low-fat)	½ cup	8
Beans, black	½ cup	8
Carnation Instant Breakfast	1 pkt	4
Cheese (low fat)	1 oz.	8
Cheese (Mozzarella)	1 pce	9
Chicken (boneless, skinless)	3 oz.	21
Chicken salad (low-fat)	½ cup	15
Chickpeas	½ cup	6
Chili	1 cup	16
Cod (baked)	3 oz.	20
Cottage cheese (low-fat)	½ cup	14
Crab (canned)	3 oz.	17
Egg	1 large	6
Flounder (cooked)	3 oz.	21
Halibut (cooked)	3 oz.	21
Lentils	½ cup	9
Lima beans (canned)	½ cup	6

FOOD ITEM	SERVING SIZE	AMOUNT OF PROTEIN (GRAM)
Lobster (cooked)	½ cup	15
Milk (skim)	½ cup	4
Milk, soy	½ cup	4
Milk, nonfat dry	1/3 cup	8
Mussels (cooked)	3 oz.	20
Navy beans (cooked)	½ cup	20
Oatmeal	1 pkt	8
Peanut butter (whipped)	2 Tbs	6
PB2 (peanut butter powder)	2 Tbs	5
Peas – split (cooked)	½ cup	8
Pinto beans (cooked)	½ cup	5
Pudding (sugar-free)	½ cup	4
Salmon (canned, pink)	3 oz.	17
Sausage pattie	1 pattie	10
Scallops	2 large	6
Snack bar	1 bar	10
Soybeans (cooked)	½ cup	15
Soybeans (dry roasted)	½ cup	34

FOOD ITEM	SERVING SIZE	AMOUNT OF PROTEIN (GRAM)
Trout (baked)	3 oz.	23
Tuna	3 oz.	25
Tuna (canned, water packed)	2 oz.	12
Turkey bologna	3 oz.	12
Turkey breast – thin sliced	3 oz.	20
Turkey breast	3 oz.	21
Turkey – ground (cooked)	3 oz.	20
Turkey – canned w/ broth	½ can (2.5 oz.)	17
Vegetable protein burger	1 burger	13
Yogurt (light, fruit-flavored)	4 oz. (½ cup)	4
Yogurt (light, Greek)	6 oz.	12
Veggie Burger (mushroom or veggie based)	1 patty	6
Vegetable Protein burger	1 patty	13

Gluten

Gluten is a protein found in many grains such as wheat, barley and rye. Gluten is common in foods such as bread, pasta and cereal; it does not provide an essential nutrient. Gluten in people with celiac disease can trigger an immune reaction that cause body to attack its own bowel tissue causing symptoms such as bloating, diarrhea and cramping and abdominal pain. Celiac disease is an autoimmune genetic disease that affects one percent of population in the United States. It is diagnosed by blood test identifying celiac disease antibody. Although celiac disease is relatively rare, there are some none celiac gluten hypersensitivity population that may benefit from gluten free diet. Gluten free diet aside from being more costly, it has higher sugar and fat content and tendency toward weight gain.

Fat

Fat is the most concentrated source of energy that is essential for our nutrition. Fat calories are twice as many per gram as the calories from protein and carbohydrates. One gram of fat produces 9 calories of energy. Daily calorie intake fat should be 20 percent of total calorie intake. Fat sources consist of oil, butter and milk. There are several forms of dietary fats.

Saturated Fats

This type of fat raises the cholesterol level and increases the risk of cardiovascular disease. Sources of saturated fats are red meat, poultry, egg yolk, coconut or palm oil, butter and whole milk. Daily intake of saturated fats should not exceed 5 percent of the calories in a meal which is approximately 13 grams of saturated fat. For example, sausage, egg and cheese for breakfast can contain 16 grams of saturated fat.

Polyunsaturated Fats

Polyunsaturated fats are simply fat molecules that have more than one unsaturated fat. Oils that contain polyunsaturated fats are typically liquid at room temperature but start to turn solid when chilled. Polyunsaturated fats can be found mostly in nuts, seeds, fish, seed oils and oyster.

Trans Fats

Trans-unsaturated fatty acids are uncommon in nature but become commonly produced industrially. Examples of trans-fats, also known as vegetable fat, are margarine, Crisco and lard. These are produced through a hydrogenation process that changes the molecular binding structure. This change in the structure makes these types of trans-fats an unhealthy choice. Daily intake of trans-fats should not exceed 2 grams.

Trans Fats will increase risk of cardiovascular disease by increasing low-density lipoprotein and cholesterol levels in our body. Replacing saturated fats with polyunsaturated fats is associated with a reduced risk of cardiovascular disease.

Cholesterols

Daily dietary intake of cholesterol should not exceed 300 mg. Besides dietary forms of cholesterol, our bodies can also manufacture cholesterol as well. Some common types of food containing cholesterol are eggs and butter. Egg and cheese for breakfast can contain 260 mg of cholesterol.

Omega 3 (Fatty acid)

Omega 3 fatty acid is a polyunsaturated fatty acid that has anti-inflammatory properties. Common sources are plant oils, walnut, flaxseed oil and fish oil.

Protein, Fat and Carbohydrate Content of Different Foods

FOOD	PERCENTAGE OF PROTEIN	PERCENTAGE OF FAT	PERCENTAGE OF CARBOHYDRATE	FINAL VALUE PER 100 GRAMS (CALORIES)
Apples	0.3	0.4	14.9	64
Asparagus	2.2	0.2	3.9	26
Bacon, fat	6.2	76.0	0.7	712
Bacon, broiled	25.0	55.0	1.0	599
Beef	17.5	22.0	1.0	268
Beets, fresh	1.6	0.1	9.6	46
Bread, white	9.0	3.6	49.8	268
Butter	0.6	81.0	0.4	733
Carrots	1.2	0.3	9.3	45
Cashew nuts	19.6	47.2	26.4	609
Cheese	23.9	32.3	1.7	393
Chocolate	5.5	52.9	18.0	570
Haddock	17.2	0.3	0.5	72
Lamb	18	17.5	1.0	230
Milk, whole	3.5	3.9	4.9	69
Oatmeal, dry	14.2	7.4	68.2	369
Oranges	0.9	0.2	11.2	50
Peanuts	26.9	44.2	23.6	600

FOOD	PERCENTAGE OF PROTEIN	PERCENTAGE OF FAT	PERCENTAGE OF CARBOHYDRATE	FINAL VALUE PER 100 GRAMS (CALORIES)
Pork, ham	15.2	31.0	1.0	340
Potatoes	2.0	0.1	19.1	85
Spinach	2.3	0.3	3.2	25
Strawberries	0.8	0.6	8.1	41
Tomatoes	1.0	0.3	4.0	23
Tuna, canned	24.2	10.8	0.5	194
Walnuts	15.0	64.4	15.6	702

Micronutrients

Micronutrients include vitamins and minerals that are organic components needed in small quantities in the cell for normal metabolism and cannot be manufactured by the cell. Vitamins and minerals are essential factors in numerous biological processes in our body. Lack of vitamins and minerals causes important metabolic difficulties. Vitamins and minerals are stored in small amounts in the cell but mostly are stored in the liver. Taking daily micronutrients supplements and eating food high in vitamins and minerals are an important aspect of our diet. Complete multivitamin and mineral supplement on daily basis should be considered with every weight loss diet as well as weight loss surgery.

Vitamin A

Vitamin A is essential for normal vision, and it plays an important role in maintaining healthy skin, mucosa membrane and teeth. Vitamin A deficiency causes night blindness.

The best food sources of vitamin A are found in spinach, broccoli, carrots, squashes, sweet potatoes, cantaloupe, fish and low-fat milk.

Vitamin B1 (Thiamine)

Vitamin B1 is a coenzyme that is essential for the metabolism of carbohydrates in various organs including heart, gastrointestinal system, peripheral and central nervous system. Thiamine deficiency is known as beriberi disease, the symptoms involve central nervous system, cardiovascular and gastrointestinal system. Cardiovascular symptoms are tachycardia, cardiac dilation, respiratory distress and edema of lower extremities. Neuromuscular symptoms are muscle weakness, pain in extremities, mental confusion and encephalopathy. Gastrointestinal symptoms cause gastric dilatation, nausea, vomiting and mega colon. Thiamine has a short half-life. In chronic malnutrition a dietary deficiency of 10-20 days can result in symptoms of thiamine deficiency. This is specially seen after weight loss surgery such as sleeve gastrectomy, Roux-en-Y gastric bypass and duodenal switch. Post-surgery vitamin supplements are necessary to prevent thiamine deficiency.

Additionally, many medications can interfere with the absorption of thiamine. Medications such as anti-reflux, H2-blocker (Zantac – Pepcid) and proton pump inhibitor (Nexium, omeprazole) and long-term use of diuretic such as Lasix. Thiamine deficiency is also seen in rapid weight loss, profound vomiting and excessive use of alcohol. The best food sources of vitamin B1 are found in the pork, other lean meats, whole grains, dried beans and peas, and eggs.

Vitamin B2 (Riboflavin)

Vitamin B2 is another coenzyme essential for the metabolism of carbohydrates and protein. It has a significant role in maintenance of the integrity of skin, lips, and mucous membranes. Vitamin B2 deficiency results in dermatitis and angular cheilitis which presents as skin breakdown in both corners of mouth with inflammation of lips. The best food sources of vitamin B2 are found in milk, cheeses, liver, meats and whole grain.

Vitamin B3 (Niacin)

Niacin is the essential coenzyme for the metabolism of glucose, fat and protein. Vitamin B3 deficiency causes dermatitis known as pellagra disease.

The best food sources of vitamin B3 are found in liver, meats, chicken, dried peas and beans, nuts and whole grains.

Vitamin B6 (Pyridoxine)

Vitamin B6 is the essential coenzyme for amino acids and protein metabolism. Vitamin B6 deficiency causes seizures, dermatitis, nausea and vomiting.

The best food sources of vitamin B6 are found in beef, chicken, tuna, salmon, pork, oatmeal, bran cereal, peanuts, bananas and eggs.

Vitamin B7 (Biotin)

Biotin provides the link between carbohydrates and fat metabolism. Biotin deficiency causes anorexia, vomiting and dermatitis and hair loss.

The best food sources of vitamin B7 are found in egg yolks, liver, kidney beans and soybeans.

Vitamin B9 (Folate - Folic Acid)

Vitamin B9 is a water-soluble vitamin. Folic acid has significant role in reducing cardiovascular disease and stroke, osteopenia, depression, cognitive decline and pernicious anemia.

Folate deficiency manifests as pigmentation or ulceration of skin, nails, or oral mucosa.

The best food sources of Vitamin B9 are found in liver, dried beans, peas, spinach, broccoli, turnip greens, oranges, yeast and nuts.

Vitamin B12 (Cobalamin)

Vitamin B12 is the coenzyme necessary for protein synthesis. It is vital for blood cell formation. Vitamin B12 deficiency causes pernicious anemia known as Megaloblastic anemia.

The best food sources of vitamin B12 are found in liver, meats, eggs and milk.

Vitamin C (Ascorbic acid)

Vitamin C aids in collagen formation and wound healing. Vitamin C deficiency cause swollen gums and cracked lips.

The best food sources for vitamin C are found in citrus fruits and juices, cantaloupe, strawberries, tomatoes, potatoes, broccoli and cabbage.

Vitamin D

Vitamin D regulates the metabolism of calcium and phosphorus and is component factor for mineralization of bone. Vitamin D is in two forms, vitamin D2 that is produced from dietary intake and vitamin D3 is obtained from sun exposure. Vitamin D deficiency will increase risk of osteomalacia and bone fracture.

The best food sources of vitamin D are found in egg yolks, liver, fish liver oils and vitamin D enriched milk.

Vitamin E

Vitamin E is an antioxidant that protects the body from changes of free radicals. Free radicals are biological toxins that have the potential of damaging our cells.

The best food sources of vitamin E are found in meats, nuts, and vegetable oil. Vitamin E supplements may increase the risk of bleeding.

Vitamin K

Vitamin K contributes to blood clotting. Vitamin K deficiency will increase problem with bruising and the risk of hemorrhage.

The best food sources of vitamin K are cabbage, peas, grains, egg yolks, liver and other green leafy vegetables.

Required daily amounts of vitamins

Vitamin	**Amount**
Vitamin A	5000 IU
Thiamin (Vitamin B1)	1.5 mg
Riboflavin (Vitamin B2)	1.8 mg
Niacin (Vitamin B3)	20 mg
Pantothenic acid (Vitamin B5)	Unknown
Pyridoxine (Vitamin B6)	2 mg
Folic acid (Vitamin B9)	0.4 mg
Ascorbic acid (Vitamin C)	45 mg
Vitamin D	400 IU
Vitamin E	15 IU
Vitamin K	40 µg

Calcium

Calcium is the essential component in the structural formation of bones and teeth. It contributes to blood clotting, muscle and nerve function. Calcium deficiency causes bone deformities. Calcium supplement should be considered with any weight loss diet and after weight loss surgery.

The best food sources of Calcium are found in milk, cheese, yogurt, salmon, sardines and mustard greens.

Phosphorus

Phosphorus is the essential component in combination with calcium necessary for the structural formation of bone and teeth. Phosphorus deficiency causes bone loss, weakness and anorexia.

The best food sources of Phosphorus are found in meats, milk, cheeses, cereals, nuts, dried beans and peas.

Magnesium

Magnesium is the necessary coenzyme in combination with carbohydrates and protein metabolism. It is also another essential component in the structural formation of bones and teeth. Magnesium deficiency cause behavioral problems and convulsions.

The best food sources of Magnesium are found in cashews, garbanzo beans, peanut butter, spinach, oatmeal and milk.

Sodium

Sodium helps maintain the right balance of fluid in our body, helps transmit nerve impulses, and influences the contraction and relaxation of muscles. Too much sodium can be harmful and can result in high blood pressure and fluid retention. Most of sodium in our diet comes from salt, soups, luncheon meats and frozen foods.

Potassium

Potassium is a vital mineral in our body, which is necessary for normal function of the heart, the nervous system and all muscles. Daily intake of potassium is 2000-4000 mg. Potassium deficiency may cause high blood pressure. Excess potassium is excreted by the kidneys. Individuals with kidney disease should limit their potassium intake. High levels of potassium in blood can cause irregular heart beat that can be potentially dangerous.

Best food sources of potassium are found in bananas, cantaloupe, kiwi, watermelon, avocado, sweet potato, yogurt, red meat, fish and chicken.

Iron

Iron is the major component of hemoglobin and myoglobin. Iron is essential during the growth period. Iron deficiency cause anemia and fatigue. Iron deficiency can be caused from low dietary intake or loss of iron during menstruation in women and blood loss. Women of premenopausal age have increased risk of iron deficiency and anemia. Additional iron supplement and folic acid should be taken daily.

The best food sources of iron are found in the liver, beef, chicken, dried beans and peas, whole grains and cereals, collard and turnip greens. Iron supplement should be taken in divided doses.

Zinc

Zinc is a mineral that plays an important role in nucleic acid metabolism, gene regulation, immune functions, hormone activity, lipid, protein metabolism, cell growth, vision and wound healing.

Copper

Copper is an essential trace mineral that act as an antioxidant. It is involved in the synthesis of pigment of melanin, connective tissue proteins, collagen and elastin.

Required daily amounts of minerals

Mineral	Amount
Sodium	3.0 g
Potassium	1.0 g
Chloride	3.5 g
Calcium	1.2 g
Phosphorus	1.2 g
Iron	18 mg
Iodine	150.0 µg
Magnesium	0.4 g
Cobalt	Unknown
Copper	900 mcg
Manganese	Unknown
Zinc	15 mg

Fiber and prebiotic

Dietary fiber is bulk and roughage that is necessary for colon function preventing constipation. Prebiotics are essential in maintaining intestinal microbiota and probiotic health. There are two types of fibers, insoluble and soluble.

Insoluble fiber

This form of fiber does not dissolve in water, it absorbs water and does not get absorbed in our body, but it helps with constipation and prevents development of diverticulosis and it may help sweep certain toxins.

Best food sources of insoluble fibers are in whole grain, corn, nuts and seeds, apple, banana and green vegetables.

Soluble fiber

Soluble fibers are digested and used as food by the good bacteria in colon.

Best food sources of soluble fibers are fruits, apples, bananas, pears plums and oat.

Water

Water is one of the most important elements of our nutrition. It is the most abundant compound in the human body. In fact, up to 75 percent of our body's weight is made of water. It plays a key role in the digestion, absorption, transportation and use of nutrient. Water sustains the right environment for our cells in the body. It also removes our metabolic waste product and toxins through kidneys. Adequate daily water intake is essential for our health. Inadequate water intake will result in dehydration that may result in headache, fatigue, light headiness and difficulty in concentration. Average daily water intake is about 64 to 96 ounces.

Probiotics

Probiotics are live bacteria and yeast that balance our gut microbiota and play a significant role in management of many digestive diseases. They help diarrhea or irritable bowel syndrome (IBS), inflammatory bowel disease and antibiotic related diarrhea. Best sources of Probiotics are found in yogurt and other fermented foods.

Antioxidants

Oxidation is a chemical reaction that can produce free radicals, leading to a chain reaction that may damage cells. Antioxidant molecules inhibits this chain reaction. However, antioxidant dietary supplements don't improve health or prevent disease.

Many vitamins such as vitamin A, vitamin C and vitamin E have antioxidant effects.

Herbs

Herbs have aromatic properties used for flavoring and garnishing foods and have effect on our metabolism.

Basil. Helps gastrointestinal gas and relieves stomach upsets.

Cinnamon. Helps lower blood sugar and helps lower blood pressure.

Rosemary. Has anti-oxidant effect.

Mint. Helps upset stomach and can ease hiccups.

Oregano. Helps soothe stomach muscles.

Cayenne. Helps heart muscle.

Fenugreek. Helps flush out harmful toxins.

Fennel. Can reduce bad breath and body odor.

Clove. Has antimicrobial effect.

Sage. Has antiseptic and antibiotic effect.

Thyme. Relaxes respiratory muscles.

Turmeric. Has anti-cancer effect.

Garlic. Is a natural antiseptic.

Ginger. Is an anti-nausea remedy.

Black pepper. Helps relieve indigestion.

Dill. Treat heartburn, colic and gas.

* * *

Chapter 10
Developing healthy dietary habits

Being overweight or obese is an ongoing and chronic problem that is not likely to be corrected by a diet for the long term. Diets have been in existence for centuries. They have a cyclic popularity, every 2-3 years a new diet becomes popular and after a while when the temporary effect of these diets fades away everyone goes back to their old eating habits and gain their weight back, then look for another new popular diet to try again. In fact, there are over 2000 weight loss diets. The basic problem with diets is that each diet will have a list of recommended food items to eat that most likely are not consistent with what we would normally eat. We will go along and follow the diet for a while, but will become bored with it. It will get old and not satisfying. Finally, old eating habits and cravings will come back and we will gain back the weight we lost.

In order to lose weight and maintain a healthy weight in the long term, we must learn and practice proper dietary habits. There are three aspects to our eating habits that determine our daily calorie intake. These three aspects are what I call **F.A.T.** to easily remember.

F – Stands for **Frequency** of eating in 24 hours.

A – Stands for **Amount** of food for each meal both in portion and calorie content.

T – Stands for **Type** of food we eat.

Frequency: Basic healthy eating habits consist of only two or three meals per day. No snaking. **There is no such thing as a healthy snack.**

Amount: We should limit our calorie intake to 1200 calories per day and pay proper attention to portion sizing. Each meal should be around 400 calories if we eat three meals a day, and 600 calories if we eat two times a day.

Type: A healthy meal is high in protein, low in carbohydrates and fat, and high in fiber.

What is the best diet? The best diet is the healthy one that we design for ourselves.

First, let's make a list of our favorite foods for breakfast, lunch and dinner.

Second, remove all high calorie food from our list.

List of high calorie food to avoid:

- Sugar (we can use artificial and natural sweeteners like truvia, stevia and sucralose)
- Candy, cookies, cake, donuts, pies, ice cream, sweetened fruit and frozen yogurt. Sherbet/sorbet, milk shakes, chocolate milk, pudding and sweetened gelatin desserts
- Chocolate
- Crackers
- Potato chips, potatoes, French fries, mashed potatoes and tater tots
- Popcorn
- Peanuts (peanut butter), almonds, cashews, pistachios and sunflower seeds
- White rice and brown rice
- Pastas and noodles
- Cereals of any kind, oatmeal and grits
- Fruit juices like orange juice, apple juice, cranberry juice and grape juice. Jellies/jams and candied fruits or dried fruits. Canned or frozen fruit in heavy syrup
- Minimize bread including wheat bread and tortillas

- Sodas or sugary drinks, sports drinks or energy drinks
- Avoid some fruits as they contain natural sugars and are extremely high in calories like watermelon, cantaloupes and bananas
- Avoid meal supplements or shakes that have excessive carbohydrates and sugar in them
- Honey, syrup and molasses

Third, search and determine portion sizing and calorie content of our favorite food list. Choose, mix and match 400 calorie per meal. For instance:

4 ounces of grilled chicken breast has 187 calories.

4 ounces of tuna has 209 calories.

One cup of tomato soup has 72 calories.

One boiled egg has 78 calories.

One cup of fat free yogurt has 95 calories.

So, with very little effort and some homework we can create our favorite diet plan that is nutritional, satisfying and sustainable. So far, our own diet is the best diet.

Healthy eating habits require timely regular meals. We need to practice chewing food thoroughly. Allow 20 minutes to eat each meal, eat slowly and sit down to eat, do not watch TV, do not use the computer, a handheld device or phone during mealtime. We must try to avoid eating food due to boredom or stress. We must avoid consumption of fast food. Also eliminate the consumption of sugary drinks and eliminate high fructose, corn syrup, high fat, high sodium and processed food. We must avoid fruit juices and high fructose fruits. Add dietary fiber such as vegetables and salad. We must avoid going to the break room where snacks are provided and avoid grazing because that will result in loss of control of our eating habit. It is important to drink one glass of water or other 0 calorie beverage before each meal. This will make us feel full faster and we will eat

Nutrition Facts	
8 servings per container	
Serving size	**3/4 cup (28g)**
Amount per serving	
Calories	**140**
	% Daily Value*
Total Fat 1.5g	**2%**
Saturated Fat 0g	**0%**
Trans Fat 0g	
Polyunsaturated Fat 0.5g	
Monounsaturated Fat 0.5g	
Cholesterol 0mg	**0%**
Sodium 160mg	**7%**
Fluoride 0mg	
Total Carbohydrate 22g	**8%**
Dietary Fiber 2g	**7%**
Soluble Fiber <1g	
Insoluble Fiber 1g	
Total Sugars 9g	
Includes 8g Added Sugars	**16%**
Protein 9g	**18%**
Vitamin D 2mcg (80 IU)	10%
Calcium 130mg	10%
Iron 4.5mg	25%
Potassium 110mg	2%
Vitamin A 90mcg	10%
Vitamin C 9mg	10%
Vitamin B_6 0.4mg	25%
Folate 200mcg DFE (120mcg folic acid)	50%
Vitamin B_{12} 0.6mcg	25%
Phosphorus 100mg	8%
Magnesium 25mg	6%
Zinc 3mg	25%

* The % Daily Value (DV) tells you how much a nutrient in a serving of food contributes to a daily diet. 2,000 calories a day is used for general nutrition advice.

Calories per gram:
Fat 9 • Carbohydrate 4 • Protein 4

less. We don't need to eat till we feel full, we need to practice to stop eating before we get full.

It is important to understand and determine nutritional contents of the foods we eat. We need to pay attention to the nutritional labeling of foods. When the label is used correctly it can guide us to choose proper type of food and appropriate calorie content. Many times, the labeling can be misleading and confusing, so we must learn to look for proper information.

Serving size. The Nutritional Facts on the food label are based on a serving size. The package may contain several serving sizes 2-3 or even 8 serving sizes. Usually serving sizes are described by cup, ounces etc. The purpose of serving size is to provide what is an appropriate amount of food to consume and not to exceed more than one serving size. If we don't pay attention to serving size of the package and don't realize how many serving sizes are in the package, we may consume more food than what we thought we have.

Calories. The calorie content is given per one serving size. For instance, if the calorie content of Nutrition label is 140 calories per serving size and there are 8 serving sizes per package then the content equal 1120 calories.

Calories from fat. It is important that we focus on the type of fat content in our food and not only the total fat. As we must limit our daily intake of Saturated fats and avoid Trans-fats.

Carbohydrates.

Simple carbohydrates such as sugar must be closely monitored, and we need to be aware that some products contain added sugars. We can see how much total sugar is in the product and whether it comes naturally or if it was added. For example, light yogurt contains sugar naturally from lactose, but we must read the Nutritional label and see if any sugar was added.

Protein content.

Protein is the most essential and efficient source of energy due to its many benefits. We must always look for high-protein foods.

Essential nutrients.

Micronutrients are essential in our diet; therefore, it is important that we monitor our daily intake of these components. The Nutritional label lists the percentage of daily required micronutrients.

* * *

Mindful eating habits require training and practice. It is about developing a new relationship with food and dealing with fullness and hunger. It is about choice, and the power of control over eating habits. Mindful eating habits are permanent changes which will require practice and developing discipline. These are the foundation of a successful weight loss process for medical or surgical weight loss.

We learn to develop a greater sense of control of overeating and learn to deal with hunger and fullness. Learn to increase tolerance to difficult and negative emotions that triggers food comfort. We also need to learn to deal with family or other caregiver that enables us and continue to practice mindful eating habits.

Usually, it takes practice of three to six months of mindful eating habits to gain full control of eating disorders.

Here is what I recommend to my patients. Every night before going to bed practice to look back and review our behavior, not only regarding our eating habits, but everything that went on all day, school, work, family, friends and coworkers. Review everything and see where we made mistakes. Learn from the mistakes we made, and try not to make those mistakes tomorrow, and tomorrow will be a better day. Remember smart people learn from other people's mistakes, but we should be able to learn from our own mistakes.

* * *

Chapter 11
Helpful recipes

List of zero calorie beverages

- Water
- Flavored water, add cool aid or crystal lite
- Regular coffee
- Decaffeinated coffee
- Black hot tea
- Flavored hot tea
- Green hot tea
- Unsweetened iced tea
- Fresh squeezed lemonade (no sugar) add artificial sweetener

You may add artificial sweetener to beverage of choice. Daily fluid intake must be 64-96 ounces.

List of other beverages

- Skim milk 6 oz (61 calories)
- Low fat milk 6 oz (74 calories)
- Almond milk 6 oz (47 calories)
- Sugar free creamer 15 calories/15 ml (tablespoon)

Choose your beverages; make sure you take a glass of your favorite beverage before each meal.

Low calorie steamed vegetable

You can have steamed vegetables with each meal. Choose any single vegetable or combine and mix your favorite one (one cup serving size is less than 120 calories).

Chop and mix vegetables of your choice add fresh ground pepper, lime or lemon juice. Boil in water until steams and water evaporates, add your favorite spices.

- Diced broccoli
- Diced cauliflower
- Chopped cabbage
- Spinach
- Diced okra
- Chopped green, yellow or red bell pepper
- Diced mushroom
- Sliced tomatoes
- Sliced white onion
- Sliced carrots
- Sliced yellow squash

Cucumber yogurt salad less than 100 calories per serving

You can have yogurt salad for lunch or dinner.

- One cup of fat free Greek yogurt
- On cucumber diced
- 2 cloves of crushed shallots
- Two tablespoons of dill weed
- One teaspoon of dry mint
- Fresh ground pepper

Mix and chill in refrigerator.

High protein meal

At least 2 meals per day must contain high protein that is **grilled** or **baked** or **broiled**.

Meat

- 4 ounces of lean stake (162 calories)
- 4 ounces of lean pork (274 calories)
- 4 ounces of lean lamb (234 calories)
- 4 ounces of lean ground beef (284 calories)

Poultry

- 4 ounces of skinless chicken (187 calories)
- 4 ounces of skinless turkey breast (214 calories)
- 4 ounces of lean ground turkey (120 calories)
- 4 ounces of fresh deli diced turkey (216 calories)
- 4 ounces of deli sliced ham (203 calories)

Fish

- 4 ounces of cod (112 calories)
- 4 ounces of tilapia (202 calories)
- 4 ounces of salmon (181 calories)
- 4 ounces of catfish (181 calories)
- 4 ounces of water packed tuna (80 calories)
- 4 ounces of swordfish (195 calories)
- 4 ounces of flounder (192 calories)
- 4 ounces of trout (192 calories)
- 4 ounces of Mahi mahi (198 calories)
- 4 ounces of Ahi tuna (120 calories)
- 4 ounces of grouper (134 calories)

Shellfish

- 4 ounces of crab meat (116 calories)
- 4 ounces of scallops (126 calories)
- 4 ounces of shrimp (100 calories)
- 4 ounces of lobster (101 calories)
- 4 ounces of clams (140 calories)

Low calorie bowl of fresh salad

Mix and toss in salad bowl and chill and add one serving of protein.

Choose and combine any item for small salad bowl:

- Chopped romaine lettuce
- Chopped iceberg lettuce
- Spring mix
- Baby spinach
- Kale
- Diced fresh broccoli
- Diced fresh cucumber
- Diced fresh mushroom
- Diced radishes
- Diced tomato
- Diced tomatoes
- Sliced or shredded carrots
- Chopped celery
- Chopped fresh parsley
- Chopped fresh cilantro
- Chopped pickles
- Chopped green, yellow or red bell pepper
- Sliced onions
- Chopped onion
- Diced onion
- Diced black olives
- Diced green olives
- Freshly chopped mint
- Sliced avocado

Add one item of protein less than 400 calories per serving. Combine and mix any of your favorite items in salad bowl, add fresh ground pepper, add 2 tablespoon of parmesan cheese, toss and chill use lemon and lime juice and balsamic vinegar.

Choose for each meal one high protein addition to your salad:

- 2 chopped boiled eggs (156 calories)
- 4 ounces of water packed tuna (80 calories)
- 4 ounces of sliced chicken (broiled, baked or grilled)
- 4 ounces of sliced tuna meat (214 calories)
- 4 ounces of fat free cottage cheese (80 calories)
- 3 ounces of fish filet

Spinach yogurt salad less than 100 calories per serving

- One cup of cooked diced spinach
- One cup of fat free yogurt
- Black pepper
- One tablespoon of garlic powder
- One teaspoon of onion powder
- May add other herbs of your choice

Mix and chill in refrigerator.

Breakfast

- Two boiled eggs or poached or scrambled (156 calories)
- Three ounces of fat free cottage cheese (80 calories)
- One cup of fat free yogurt (130 calories)

Simple egg omelet

- Two eggs
- One tablespoon of fat free cheese
- Two tablespoons of fat free milk
- Add fresh ground pepper or other spices of your choice like cumin

Scramble and cook in nonstick pan or in oven.

Turkey bacon omelet

- Two eggs
- One tablespoon of fat free cheese
- Two tablespoons of fat free milk
- Two slices of turkey bacon diced in small pieces
- Add fresh ground pepper and spices of your choice, like curry, cumin, cinnamon, vanilla or garlic powder

Mix in bowl and cook in nonstick pan while scrambling it or cook in oven.

Omelet

- Two eggs
- ¼ cup of chopped onion
- ¼ cup of cream peas cooked or canned fresh
- ¼ cup of chopped mushrooms (fresh or canned)
- ¼ cup of chopped tomatoes
- One tablespoon of low-fat cottage cheese, parmesan cheese or shredded cheddar cheese
- Add dash or black pepper or other species

Stir and mix with two eggs and place in pan. Cook for 20 minutes in 200-degree oven.

Vegetable omelet

- Two eggs
- One bunch of celery chopped or blended

- One bunch of leaks chopped or blended
- ¼ cup of spinach chopped
- Two eggs mixed
- One tablespoon of shredded low-fat cheese
- Add dash
- Ground pepper

Mix and stir with two eggs and place in pan. Cook for 20 minutes in 200-degree oven.

Tomato omelet

- Two eggs
- ½ cup of crashed tomatoes
- Two tablespoons of fat free cheese
- Two tablespoons of fat free milk
- Two eggs
- One tablespoon of bread crumbs
- One tablespoon of baking soda
- Black pepper
- Add spices of your choice like dash, curry, cumin, cinnamon, vanilla or garlic powder.

Mix and cook for 20 minutes in 200-degree oven.

Spinach omelet

- Two eggs
- One cup of cooked diced spinach
- Two eggs
- Two tablespoons of fat free cheese
- Two tablespoons of fat free milk
- One tablespoon of baking soda
- Add fresh ground pepper
- Add any spice of your choice like curry, cumin, cinnamon, vanilla or garlic powder

Stir and mix and place in a pan. Cook for 20 minutes in 200-degree oven.

Mixed vegetable omelet

- Chose and combine any vegetable of your choice
- ¼ cup of diced celery

- ¼ cup of diced leak
- ¼ cup of white onion
- Add two eggs
- Two tablespoons of fat free cheese
- Two tablespoons of fat free milk
- One tablespoon of bread crumb
- One tablespoon of baking soda
- Add fresh ground black pepper
- Add spices of your choice, dash, curry, cumin, cinnamon, vanilla or garlic powder

Stir and mix and place in a pan and cook for 20 minutes in 200-degree oven.

Stuffed cabbage

- 4 ounces of fat free ground meat
- 4 ounces of chopped vegetables (add leak, cilantro or parsley)
- 2 ounces of dirty rice
- One tablespoon of curry
- One tablespoon of cumin
- One egg
- One teaspoon of freshly ground black pepper

Mix in bowl. Peel cabbage leaves boiled in water to soften it. Take golf ball sized of meat and vegetable mix. Place in cabbage and wrap cabbage over it and stack up in cooking pan. Add one can of tomato paste mixed with water allow the packed cabbage cook for 30 minutes.

Cup of soup

- Chicken soup (70 calories)
- Cream of broccoli (80 calories)
- Cream of mushrooms (90 calories)
- Tomato, mushroom and cabbage soup (85 calories)
- 4 ounces of fat free cottage cheese (80 calories)
- ½ grapefruit (41 calories)

* * *

Chapter 12

Exercise for individuals with limited mobility

1. **Breathing exercise**
   Take a slow deep breath in and hold it for as long as you can, then exhale. Repeat 10 times at least 3 times a day and each time try to take a deeper breath.

2. **Neck exercise**
   A) Slowly bring your chin to your chest and hold for 2 second then raise your head all the way back and hold it for 3 seconds. Repeat 20 times, three times a day.

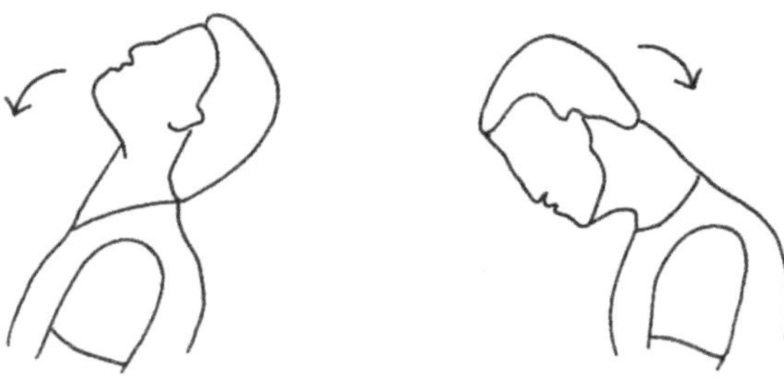

   B) Slowly turn your head to the right then slowly turn it to the left. Repeat 20 times, three times a day.

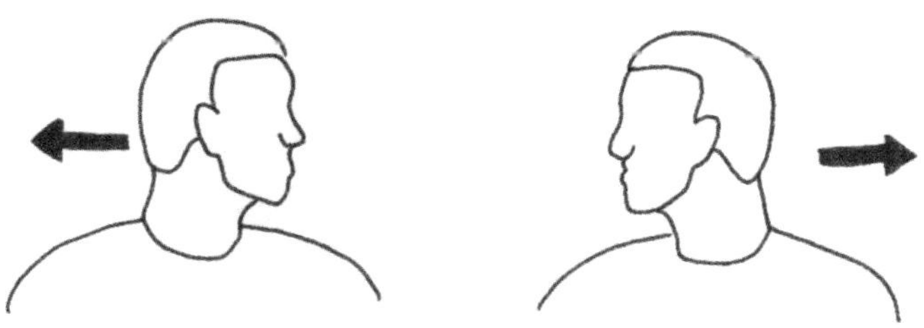

C) Slowly turn your head side to side bend your neck moving your ear toward your shoulder. Repeat 20 times, three times a day.

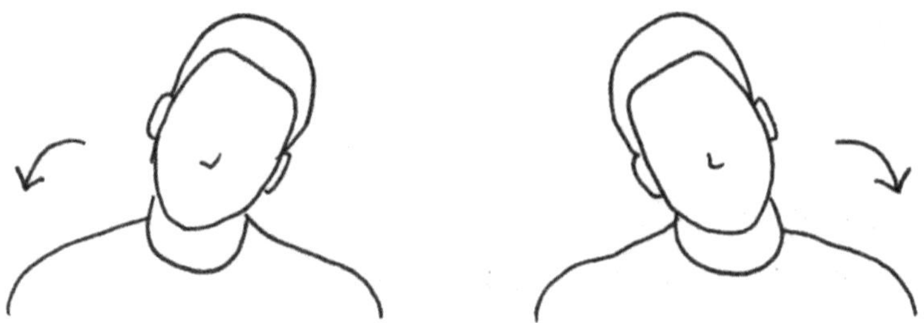

3. Shoulder exercise

A) Sitting or standing with both arms on your side lift both shoulders up toward your ears and then back down. Repeat 20 times, 3 times a day.

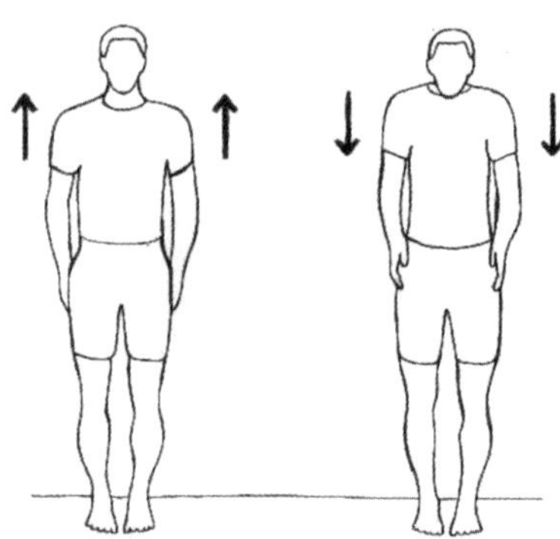

B) With your arms at your side raise your arms away from your body up to level of your shoulder then back down to your side. Repeat 20 times, three times a day.

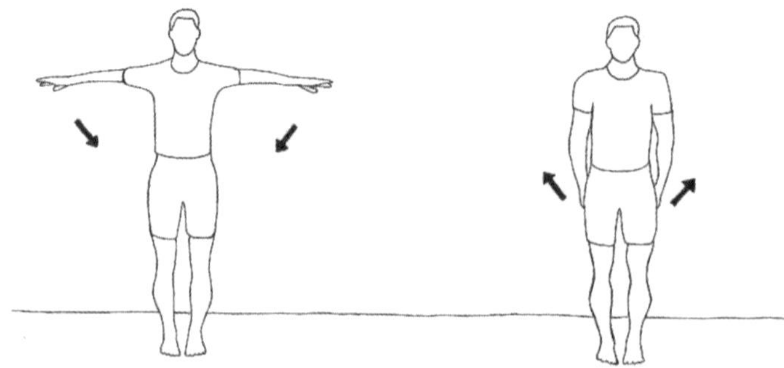

C) With your arms to your side raise one arm straight up in front of you so your arm is by your ear then move back down. While moving one arm down raise the other arm up. Repeat 20 times, three times a day.

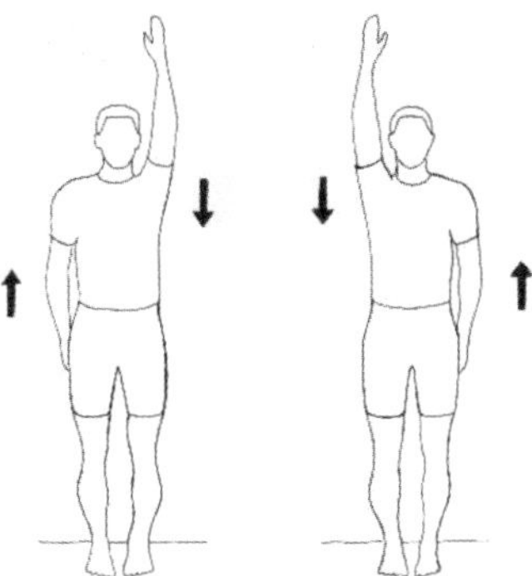

D) With your arms at your side raise your arms away from your body up to straight so your arms are near your ears and your hands touch each other above your head and then bring your arm back down. Repeat 20 times, three times a day.

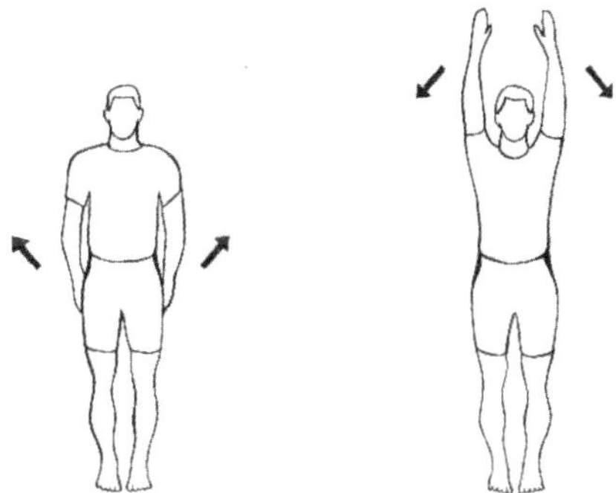

E) Bend your elbows and put your hands as fist together and raise your elbows at the level of your shoulders. Then push your elbows as far back as you can at the level of shoulders and spread your hands. Then bring your hands back together and keep your chest forward. Repeat 20 times, three times a day.

F) With your arms at your side raise your arms away from your body up to level of your shoulder then rotate your arms clockwise so your hand will draw a circle about a large dinner plate, repeat 20 times. Then do the same rotate your arm but this time counterclockwise 20 more times. Repeat three times a day.

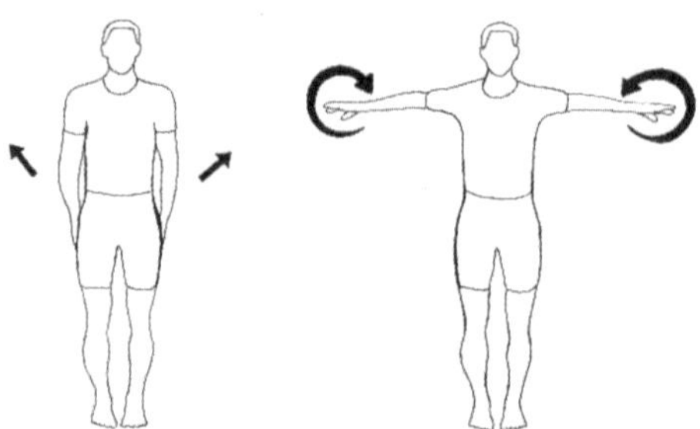

4. Arm exercise

A) With your arms at your side bend your elbow all the way so your hand is near your shoulder then straighten your elbow. Repeat 20 times three times a day. Next try this with some weight or a can of food.

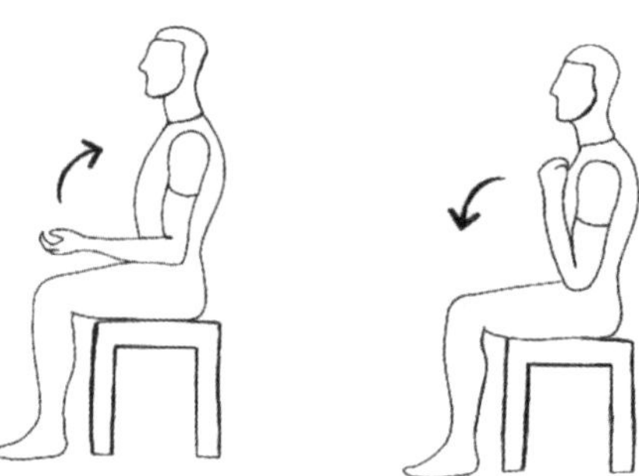

B) Hold your arms to your side with the elbows 90 degree then turn your palm toward floor and then ceiling. Repeat 20 times, three times a day.

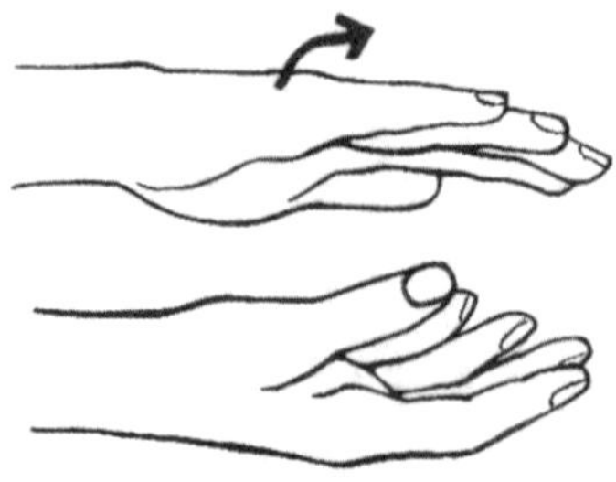

5. **Hand exercise**

A) Open and close your hands 20 times, three times a day.

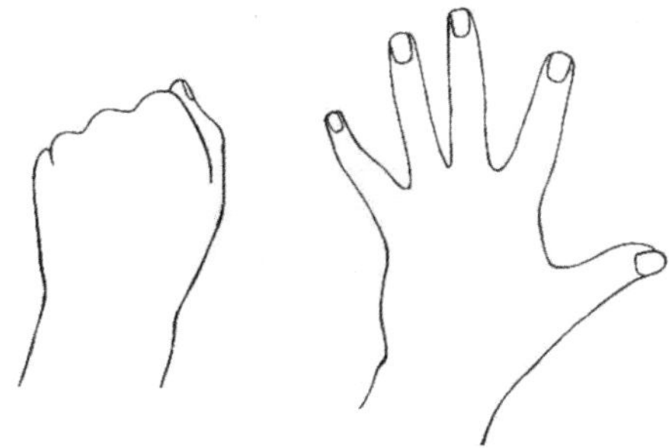

B) Place your forearm on a table with your hand off the edge with the palm down, then move your hand up and down. Repeat 20 times each hand, three times a day.

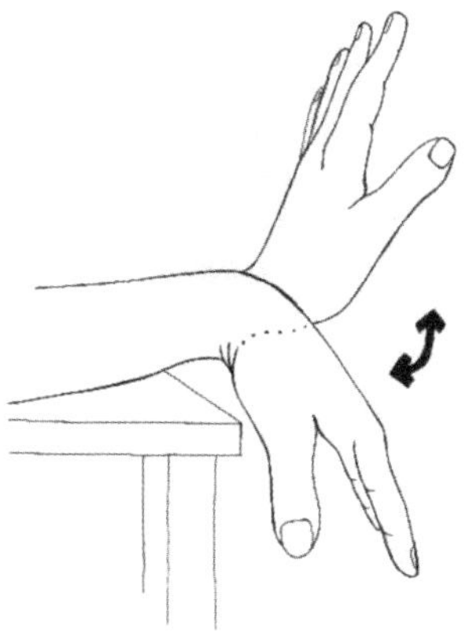

6. **Leg exercise**

A) Sitting in chair march in place move your feet up and down. Repeat 30 times, three times a day.

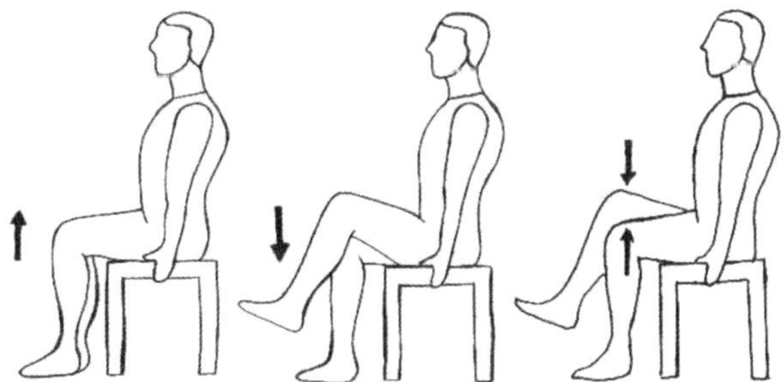

B) Sitting in a chair spread your knees apart as far as you can and then bring them together. Repeat 20 times, three times a day.

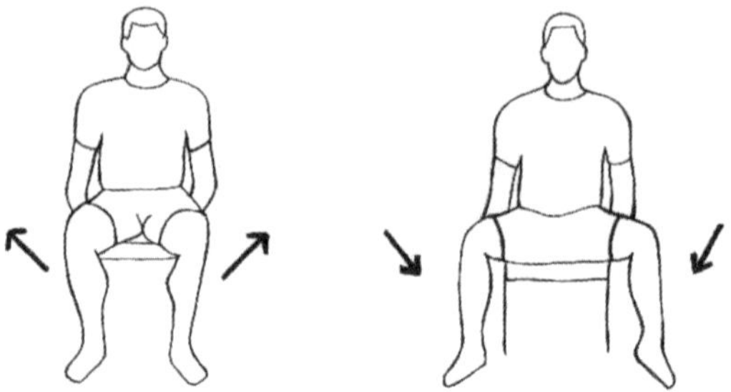

C) Sitting in a chair kick one leg up to straighten your knee then bring it down, do the other leg next. Repeat 20 times, three times a day.

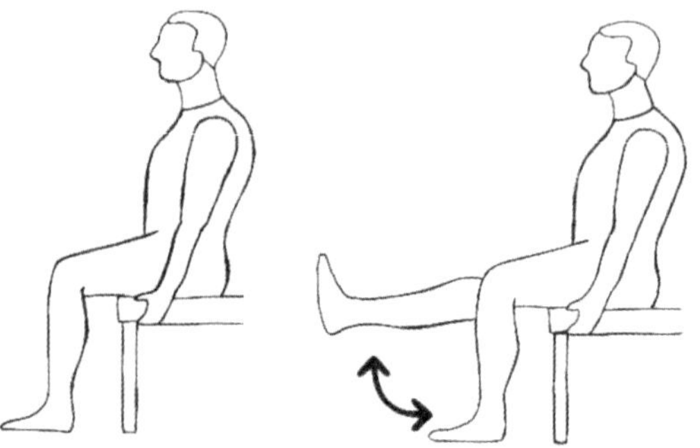

D) With your heel on the floor move your foot up and down. Repeat 20 times each foot, three times a day.

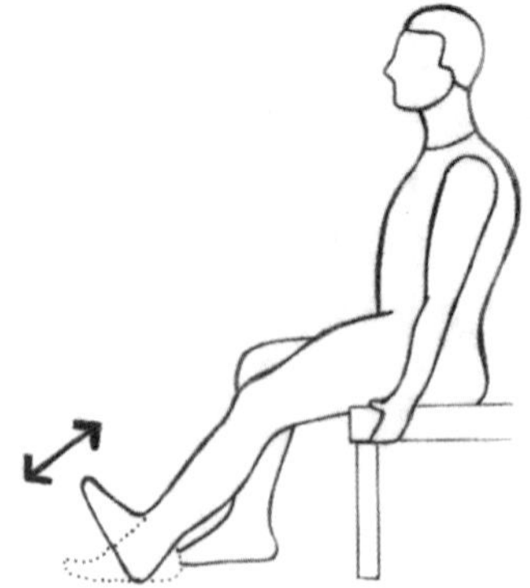

E) Laying on your back on the floor or in the bed raise your leg straight up as far as you can then put it down and do the same with other leg. Repeat 20 times, three times a day.

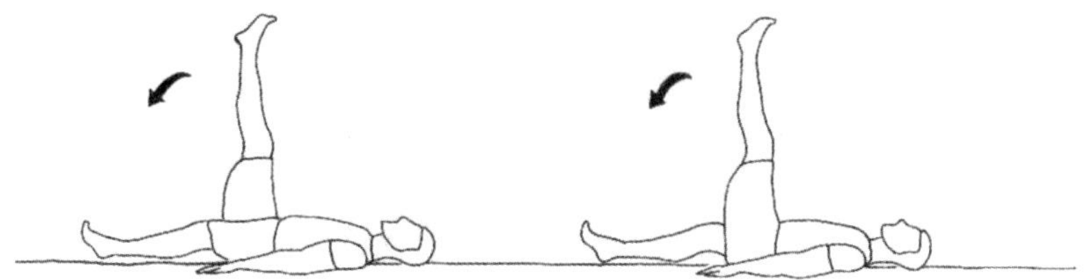

F) Laying on your back on the floor or in the bed raise one leg and bend your knee and bring your knee toward your chest as far as you can then put your leg down and do the same with your other leg. Repeat 20 times, three times a day.

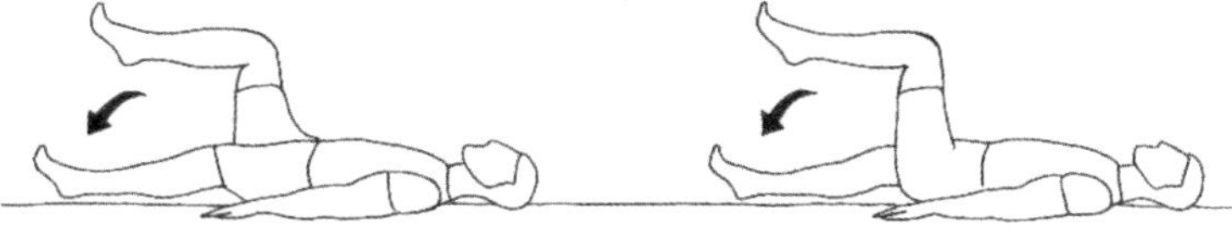

7. **Torso exercise**

   A) Standing up straight put your feet apart with your arms on your side turn your upper body and torso to the right and then to the left. Repeat 20 times, three times a day.

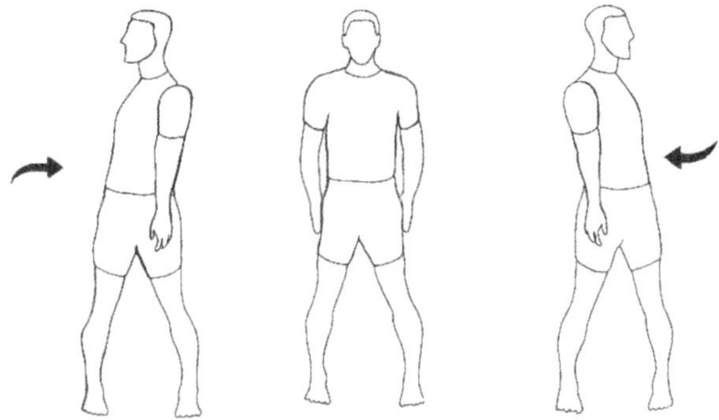

B) Standing up with your feet together bend forward and try to touch your toes with your finger then raise up straight. Repeat 20 times, three times a day.

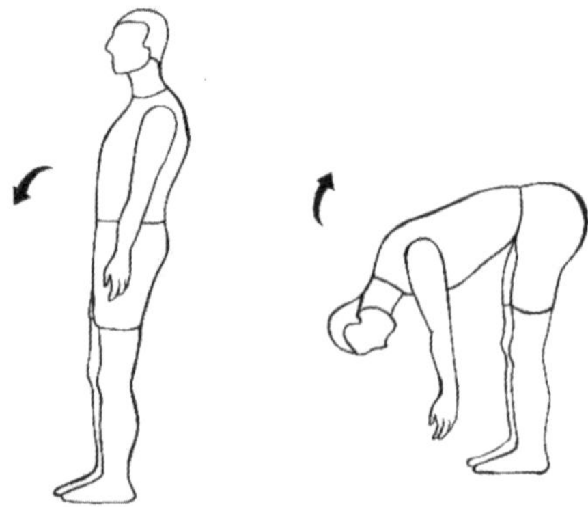

C) Standing up straight raise one arm up and bend your torso to the other side as far as you can then bring the arm down and raise the other arm and bend your torso to opposite site. Repeat 20 times, three times a day.

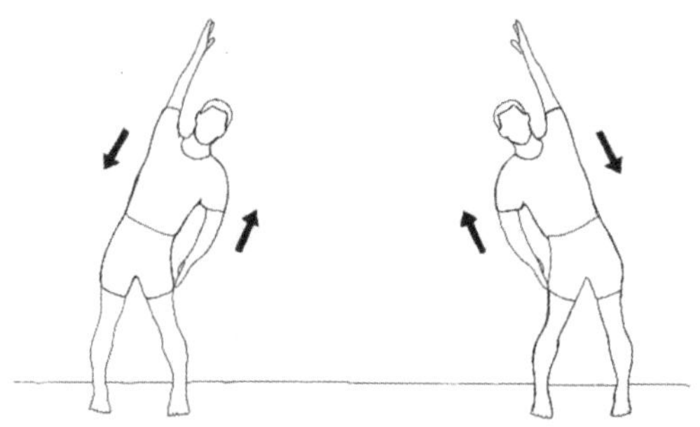

* * *

Chapter 13
Dysfunctional eating disorder

One of the most common forms of maladaptive eating disorder that results in obesity is binge eating. This condition is associated with loss of self-control of eating and despite the negative consequences the individual eats until is uncomfortably full. Binge eating can be the most difficult condition to be able to correct.

One form of binge eating is night eating syndrome when individual does not eat early in the day but has uncontrollable eating habit at night. Another form of maladaptive eating disorder is eating in absence of hunger. These individuals need to avoid food environment.

Short term medication can be used in treatment of binge eating in adults. One of such medication that is commonly used is Fluoxetine (Prozac) which is an antianxiety medication. Another medication is Lisdexanfetamine (Vyvanse) which is medication used in treatment of attention deficit disorder.

Any modality of treatment of obesity whether it is medical or surgical will not have a lasting effect when dysfunctional eating behaviors are not properly addressed. While weight loss surgery is a powerful tool to bring awareness to the eating process and help control food intake, it will not have long term success if the eating disorder prior to the surgery has not been properly corrected. Weight loss surgery cannot always control dysfunctional eating behavior especially if eating is used as a coping mechanism. From the moment of birth, the first feeling of being fed gives the sensation of satisfaction, safety, contentment and being cared for. Therefore, it is natural that food becomes symbol of safety and contentment in our life. In the development stages of life, negative feeling can trigger emotions of coping mechanism that lead to regression and a return to symbol of safety from food. Food comfort will become a coping mechanism to deal with negative emotions.

During the development stages of life, many events such as being raised in an abusive home, parental dispute, divorce, being in a foster home, emotional, physical or sexual abuse and sometimes failure to earn parental or other family member's love can lead to emotions that trigger coping behavior and the person will turn to food for comfort. This is often seen in childhood or adolescent obesity.

Food comfort also plays a significant role in adult life. Negative emotions in adult life such as sense of inferiority and low self-esteem, failure to progress in life, sense of emptiness and self-condemnation, harsh self-criticism result in seeking for food comfort. It may also result in diminished social skills leading to a tendency of isolation and depression which is a hallmark of severe obesity. Depression can be a trigger factor for overeating and weight gain and obesity. Obesity itself can be source of depression as well. Bidirectional association between obesity and depression can result in vicious circle that is commonly seen in morbidly obese individuals. In such a case weight loss surgery will not correct such behavior and will eventually result in the resurfacing of all negative emotion that will derail any weight loss progress achieved from surgical procedure.

Extreme obesity, food comfort behavior, fear of being judged by the public and social stigma will result in seeking emotional dependency on an enabler. It is vitally important that dysfunctional eating disorders prior to weight loss surgery be properly evaluated and addressed. A psychological evaluation prior to considering weight loss surgery is necessary to address any coping mechanism that may surface after weight loss surgery.

Dysfunctional eating behavior must be recognized and well understood by both clinicians and the obese individuals. That objective is to develop a “mindful” eating habit prior to surgery. This brings awareness back into the whole eating process. It is important to implement a practice of mindful eating habits for three to six months prior to weight loss surgery. This provides the power of controlling eating habits and ensures the success of weight loss surgery.

In treatment of obesity, depression and substance abuse behavior should not be overlooked. Alcohol and tobacco such as smoking or vaping nicotine are symptoms of addictive behavior that parallel food addiction. Continued tobacco and alcohol abuse are contradictory to willingness for change to a healthy lifestyle and it is contraindication to any weight loss surgery.

* * *

Chapter 14
Management of Obesity

Obesity is defined as excess body fat. It is due to prolonged intake of excess calories. Obesity is a life-threatening disease that if it is not treated it will shorten our life expectancy by as much as 20 years.

The medical profession for a long time had done nothing to address obesity but recommend eat less and exercise more. It was only after the rate of obesity reached epidemic levels that the medical community recognized the need for intervention in addressing obesity. Obesity is a complex metabolic condition and the exact cause of it is not well understood. Genetic predisposition plays a significant role in the development of obesity; perhaps more than 85 percent of the time. Environmental factors that affect epigenetic obesity are also partially responsible for the obesity epidemic. One of these factors that affect obesity is high-calorie, highly processed food that is affordable and has addictive taste that is readily and widely available. Sedentary lifestyle of modern times and changes in gastrointestinal microbial flora seems to play a significant role in development of obesity. The modern-day stressful lifestyle, depression, psychological and emotional factors seems to play an important role in our eating habits. These multiple factors create a multidimensional situation that is complex and is not fully understood.

Because of multitude of opinions, that may be contradictory and confusing regarding the options of treatment of obesity, there is a high rate of failure and disappointing results, by both physician and obese individual. There is no consensus of opinion regarding what is considered a healthy diet. With over 2000 weight loss diets, several hundreds of weight loss medications and remedies, multiple invasive and noninvasive surgical options, yet there is no clear pathway for the treatment of obesity epidemic.

Moreover, there are national and global governmental regulations in the United States and many other countries regarding food industry that impose regulations on personal freedom of choice. Such regulatory mandates are unlikely to affect individual behaviors regarding their eating habits. Simply because such regulations do not address the core issues related to the development of the obesity epidemic and fail to recognize the problem on a large-scale. It appears they are trying to correct the problem without fully comprehending the cause. There are increasing suggestions that the global epidemic of obesity may be more related to metabolic changes involving environmental factors that affect gastrointestinal microbial flora which appear to be responsible for the drive to overeat and development of obesity cravings.

It is important to understand that obesity in many cases may not be the person's choice. Many factors impacting this disease are simply outside of person's control particularly in the severely obese individual. Stigma, prejudice and bias against severely obese individuals exist both in the general public and the medical community. The existence of such prejudices by the medical community will undermine the result of treatment.

Genetic predisposition plays a significant role in development of obesity as well as numerous environmental factors. Since genetic predisposition and environmental factors vary in every individual, there is no single solution that is going to fit all. The choices of solutions will vary depending on degree of obesity and the underlying causes.

Prolonged lifestyle changes, effective behavioral modifications, proper dietary habits and an increased physical activity are fundamental in management of obesity. However, in many cases it may not be enough to overcome obesity

Food plays a significant role in our life, but it must not control our life. Proper modification of our behavior and changing our life style will allow us to develop a new and healthier relationship with food. Although it may seem that a role of therapist is essential to achieve behavioral modifications, in many cases this can be simply self-accomplished by following my step by step guideline.

Step one: Developing the right attitude.

Attitude is everything in our life. It is one of the most important factors which determine success in our life. A good attitude can change a bad day into a better or even a great day. A bad attitude is like a broken car it will not get us anywhere unless we fix it. We must learn to keep a positive attitude at all times regardless of the circumstances in our life. Our attitude will affect our emotions which affects our behavior which affects life. We must understand that life is not fair all the time. Many things happen in our life that we may not have control over, but we must control how we react to it and strive to keep a positive attitude. Keep a smile that will not fade away no matter what happens. If we keep our face to the light and sunshine the dark shadows will always be behind us. We must not feel victims of circumstance and blame everyone and everything for what happens to us. No matter how tough things get in our life it matters how we react to it. In order to achieve our greatest potential in our life we must learn how to improve our attitude in our daily life. We must learn to assess our attitude and look back every day and assess our behavior with logic and see how we could have done better. Learn from our mistakes and our short falls so tomorrow we won't make the same mistakes and we will be prepared for a better day. A good judgment comes from experience. Experience comes from learning from the result of using bad judgment and mistakes in the past. We must strive to own a heart that does not hate. We must respect everyone but also have a sense of self-respect and have pride in what we do. We must love everyone without expecting others to love us back, that way our life will not be affected by someone else's feelings and behavior toward us.

So, in summary we must have a daily therapy session with ourselves and assess our emotions, behavior and our attitude and see how we can improve it so we will have a better day tomorrow.

Step two: Develop the desire and willingness to improve the quality of our life.

Our life is reflection of our desire and our dreams. Our dreams in our life need a goal because a dream without a goal is just a dream. We must have daily goal in our life. We must have willingness to work hard to achieve our dream. We must not be afraid to go to bed late and still get up early the next day. We must also have a weekly goal, monthly goal, yearly goal and above all a life time goal. We must train ourselves to start a day with a task and end the day with the task completed.

We must have daily check list. Make notes of the goals and tasks to be completed and at the end of the day go over check list and prepare for the next day. We must list tasks and weekly goals at the beginning of the week and check list at the end of the week.

Every month we write the goals to be accomplished during the month, and then check list at the end of the month. Each year we write goals to be completed at the end of the year check the list of goals completed. On daily basis we grade our attitude and go over our check list.

Step three: Developing proper dietary habits.

Diets have been around for a long time and have a cyclic popularity. Every 2-3 years a new diet will become popular.

There are many weight-loss diets, over two thousand have been around for years. Most of the diets in the long run are not effective in accomplishing a durable and sustainable weight loss. The problem with any diet is that it is temporary solution for a permanent problem. Everyone bites the bullet and will eat the item listed in the diet despite it is not their choice of the food. They will lose few pounds but sooner or later they will return to their old eating habits and gain the weight back. Any weight loss diet that consumes stored body fat for source of energy will result in production of ketones.

Learning proper dietary habits based on human digestive system, anatomy and physiology is a permanent change in eating habits that will help us have proper nutrition and achieve a healthy weight. This is a life style change that requires reading food labels, knowing the number of calories, daily preparation of food, keep a diary of the food consumed and keep track of weight.

Unfortunately, misdirected eating habits that are circulating around create a confusing state of information. Proper knowledge of basic nutrition (see Chapter 9) is required to be able to outline a healthy dietary habit. We must implement a plan of our dietary meals and follow a schedule to develop healthy eating habits.

The basic rules are: we eat 2 or 3 times a day, there is no snacking, there is no such thing as healthy snacks. Human anatomy and physiology are not compatible with frequent eating. Our digestive process takes 6-8 hours to be completed. We do not need to add to our food intake, our digestive system is capable of storing a sizable amount of food. Our liver can store energy for many hours or even days, so we do not need to eat frequently. Eating frequently will result in grazing and loss of control of eating habits which results in weight gain and contrary to circulating myth, it does not speed up our metabolism.

We must take time at least 20 minute per meal. No standing up eating, watching TV, phone or even using social media during meal time. We must learn to chew food thoroughly. We must have portion control and count calories for every meal 400 calories for 3 meals a day and 600 calories for two meals a day. Must check our weight weekly and record our progress. The best diet plan is the one that you design for yourself, using food you like for breakfast, lunch and dinner. Eliminate high calorie foods and then you search count calories of food per meal. Choose 400 calorie for breakfast, lunch and dinner. 1200 calorie daily is a starting point and check your weekly weight to adjust your calorie intake. We must chew food thoroughly and follow a high protein no carb diet. Carbs are unnecessary calories. We must take daily multivitamin, fiber and probiotic and learn not to snack. We must drink at least 64-96 ounces of water or any zero-calorie beverage daily.

We must implement daily physical activity. No carbonated or sugary drinks, no alcohol or tobacco use. Once a week one meal can be carbohydrates, we should be able to lose 5 percent of body weight per month. For instance, a 200-pound person should normally lose 10 pounds in a month.

Step four: Plan to increase physical activity.

Automated modern life style has brought technological advances in transportation, elevator, escalator and automated industrial devices that reduce the need for human physical activity which has resulted in a more sedentary life style. Additionally, a modern life style leaves very little or no time to exercise or perform physical activity. Daily physical activity is a significant part of life style change. Daily physical activity should be part of one's life. We must develop habits of not parking in the closest spot and take stairs when we can. We must dedicate 20-30 minute daily to physical activity to increase muscle tone and cardiovascular exercises such as brisk walks, jogging, cycling or treadmill.

Lifestyle modifications such as dietary restriction and increased physical activity are essential to achieve a healthy goal weight. However, the higher the BMI is, there is a less degree of probability that this alone will be sufficient enough to achieve such goal. Additionally, modality of treatment needs to be considered to augment our weight loss efforts such as anti-obesity medications and surgical options.

* * *

Anti-obesity medications

There are multiple anti-obesity medications commercially available. Unfortunately, anti-obesity medications are associated with high rate of adverse effects. Their long-term results are limited and often disappointing. Their temporary effect after the medication is discontinued is associated with high rate of weight gain.

Phentermine

This is a prescribed medication that was first introduced in treatment of obesity in 1959. It is the most affordable weight loss medication it induces weight loss by reducing appetite. It is used as a single dose of 37.5 mg early in day due to side effect of insomnia. It is recommended only for short term use due to adverse effect. Most common side effects are dizziness, anxiety, rapid heartbeat, increased blood pressure, insomnia, diarrhea or constipation. A lower dose form of this medication is available in individual dose of 8 mg for 3 times a day; however, it is much more costly.

Orlistat (Alli)

This is an over the counter medication available without prescription. This medication is lipase inhibitor. Lipase is a digestive enzyme that is secreted from pancreas in the gastrointestinal tract that helps break down of fat absorption in the small bowel. This medication reduces absorption of fat from food therefore has a limited effect on weight loss. This medication is approved for use in obesity in adolescent age 12-16 years. Prolonged use of this medication can result in fat soluble vitamin deficiency, such as vitamin E and vitamin D. This medication is reasonably priced and is affordable. Most common side effects are diarrhea, flatulence and leaking oily stool.

Topiramate

This is prescription medication that is a large spectrum anticonvulsive (seizures) medication that has been used in prevention of migraine headache. This medication has side effect of reducing appetite and has been used for weight loss. The FDA has approved the combination of topiramate with phentermine (Qsymia) for weight loss purposes. The combination of medication is relatively costly. Adverse effect of topiramate are dizziness, tingling, in hand and feet, restlessness, nausea, diarrhea, fatigue, depression, impaired memory and cognitive disorder. This medication currently is reasonably priced and affordable.

Lorcaserin (Belviq)

This medication will centrally reduce appetite. This medication currently is costly. Adverse effects are headache, dizziness and nausea.

Naltrexone/bupropion (Contrave)

This is a combination of two medications. Naltrexone is an opioid receptor antagonist. Bupropion is an anti-anxiety medication that is also used for smoking cessation. This combination of medication is a prescribed medication that currently is costly. It is used to reduce appetite and effect on weight loss. The most common adverse effect is nausea.

Lisdexamfetamine (Vyvanse)

This medication is used for treatment of hyperactivity disorder and attention deficit and is FDA approved for used for treatment of binge eating disorder in adults. This medication is considered class II-controlled substance due to abuse and dependency. This medication is costly.

Fluoxetine (Prozac)

This medication is an antidepressant medication that has been used in obsessive compulsive behavior and can reduce food intake. This medication is reasonably priced.

Metformin

Metformin is reasonably priced and affordable; it is the most commonly prescribed medication for treatment of diabetes. Metformin lowers blood sugar by reducing hepatic glucose production, decreases gastrointestinal glucose absorption and increases sensitivity to insulin. Metformin also will favorably change the microbiota in our gastrointestinal tract and result in creating short chain fatty acid and cause low density fatty acid and lower sugar in blood and decreases body weight. Even though this medication is not approved by the FDA for weight loss, metformin can be used 500 mg twice a day for weight loss purposes. The effect of metformin on the gastrointestinal tract causes some of gastrointestinal symptoms seen such as diarrhea, gas and abdominal pain. Starting metformin in lower dose with gradual increase dosage will provide better tolerance of this medication. Microflora of our gastrointestinal tract has significant role in our metabolism and our food intake. Changing gastrointestinal microbiota may be a promising future of developing medication for treatment of obesity.

Metformin is also used in treatment of polycystic ovarian syndrome. In polycystic ovarian syndrome the excess production of androgen results in increase insulin resistance. Adverse effects of metformin include headache, weakness, nausea, vomiting, diarrhea, abdominal pain and gas. Caution should be in using metformin in kidney disease and impaired liver function.

Insulin

The source of energy from the food is absorbed from the gastrointestinal tract in the form of glucose. Glucose will stimulate the pancreas to secrete insulin into our blood. It is a hormone that affects the metabolism of sugar and carbohydrates. Insulin plays a significant role in transporting glucose into the cells in our body for immediate use as energy. Also, insulin transports glucose into muscle and liver cells to be stored in form of glycogen to be used as source of energy between meals. The excess amount of energy from the food that cannot be stored in liver and muscle with the help of insulin will be stored in the form of fat. Impaired or lack of production of insulin from the pancreas due to inability to transport glucose in the cells will result in elevated blood sugar. This is known as type I diabetes mellitus which is treated by subcutaneous injections of insulin.

Type II diabetes mellitus is associated with normal or even higher level of secretion of insulin from pancreas but decreased insulin sensitivity and increased insulin resistance. When blood sugar is low pancreas secrets a hormone that is known as glucagon. Glucagon is a hormone that opposes the effect of insulin and converts glycogen from liver to glucose and elevates blood sugar. This is known as insulin resistance; our blood sugar is regulated by the balance between insulin and glycogen activity. Metformin is a medication that reduces blood sugar by lowing insulin resistance. Obese individuals invariably have increased level of insulin production but decreased insulin sensitivity and increased insulin resistance that results in elevated blood sugar (Type II diabetes mellitus).

Type II diabetes should not be treated with injections of insulin since they have already higher level of insulin and additional insulin will elevate the blood sugar and cause rapid weight gain. Type II diabetes in obese individual should be effectively treated by reducing insulin resistance and weight loss.

Glucagon antagonist

These are glucagon inhibitors. Mostly in form of injectable therapy that provide blood sugar control in type II diabetes and produce effective weight loss and is the preferred treatment of type II diabetes in obese individuals. The most effective way to eliminate insulin resistance is Roux-en-Y gastric bypass (RYGB) diverting passage of food from first portion of duodenum will eliminate stimulation of secreting glucagon from pancreas. Therefore, it is the most effective treatment of type II diabetes by eliminating the secretion of glucagon and insulin resistance. After RYGB we will have an uninhibited effect of insulin. For this reason, after ingestion of meal with high sugar or short chain carbohydrate result in sudden secretion of insulin that will result in drop of blood sugar that will manifest by weakness, cramps and diarrhea, this is known as dumping syndrome. For this reason, after RYGB surgery, sugar or short chain carbohydrate should not be consumed to prevent dumping syndrome.

Liraglutide (Saxenda)

Liraglutide is a glucagon antagonist that is a subcutaneous injection that promote control of glucose and reduce appetite, in addition it also lower blood pressure. This is the most expensive anti-obesity medication. Most common adverse effects are nausea, vomiting, diarrhea and dehydration. This medication is contraindicated in history of medullary thyroid carcinoma and multiple endocrine neoplasia. This medication is costly. Multiple anti-diabetic medications that are glucagon like peptide receptor agonist such as exenatide (Bydureon, Byetta, victoza are used for treatment of obesity in conjunction with type 2 diabetes).

* * *

Obesity is a complex multifactorial condition with variety of factors that play a role in its development, such as cultural, socio-economical, psychological, genetic and hormonal factors, but a key role of gastrointestinal microbial flora must not be overlooked. A future promising new treatment or prevention of obesity may come as pharmacotherapy that will effectively and favorably change gastrointestinal microbes and their function.

Anti-obesity medications have not been very effective in treatment of obesity due to their adverse effects, high cost and temporary effect while medication is used.

Life style change and behavior modification along with proper dietary habit and increased physical activity with short term usage of Anti-obesity medication can be effective treatment of overweight individuals (BMI between 25-29.9 kg/m^2) and most effective in class I obesity (BMI between 30-34.9 kg/m^2) and less effective in class II obesity (BMI between 35-39.9 kg/m^2).

This mode of therapy will not be durable in class III obesity (BMI of 40 kg/m^2 or greater) since the genetic disposition of obesity will not be effectively alter this complex metabolic disease, and surgical option will be the most effective altering their faulty metabolism. Surgical treatment results in physical limitation of food intake and reducing or eliminating hormonal pathway that control hunger and satiety.

* * *

Chapter 15
Weight loss surgery's past, present and future

The need for an effective treatment of obesity was recognized by the surgical community in the 1950's. After World War II the observation of sustained weight loss despite increased calorie intake in the patients who had lost a portion of their small bowel for various reasons, cultivated the idea of malabsorption mechanism for weight loss surgery.

A normal small bowel is approximately 20 feet long to provide adequate absorption of nutrients. A significant reduction of the small bowel length causes decreased absorption of nutrients. In the 1960's **jejunoileal bypass** was introduced as a weight loss surgical procedure. In this procedure 8 to 14 inches of proximal small bowel (jejunum) is connected to 4 to 12 inches of distal small bowel (ileum). The rest of the small bowel was then excluded from the passage of food.

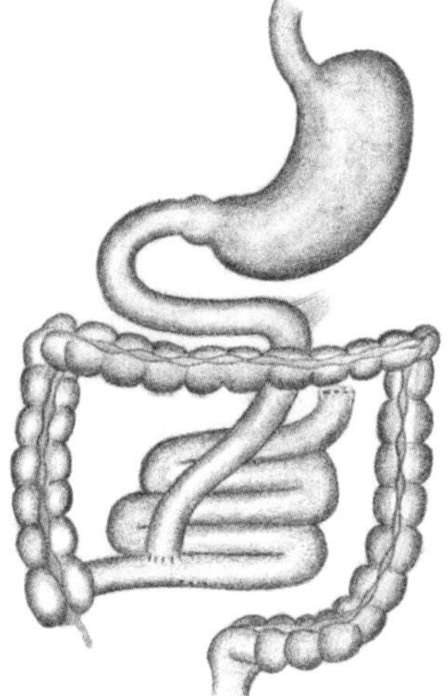

Jejunoileal bypass

Although this procedure resulted in initial weight loss, it had high complications rates and was associated with profound diarrhea, overgrowth of bacteria and toxins in bypassed segment of small bowel with development of sepsis and joint inflammation. In addition, this procedure resulted in protein calorie malnutrition, kidney stones and liver failure. This procedure was eventually abandoned and was no longer performed because of these serious complications. After that the pendulum of weight loss surgery swung from malabsorptive procedures to restrictive procedures.

In 1969 the first **gastric bypass** surgery was performed as a weight loss procedure. Initially, this procedure included creating a small proximal gastric pouch and connecting it to the small intestine. This technique later was perfected to **Roux-en-Y gastric bypass**, that provides both restrictive and malabsorption mechanisms. This procedure is reversible, and it has stood the test of time and still remains as the gold standard and most effective weight loss procedure.

Roux-en-Y gastric bypass initially was performed via an open approach and currently is performed laparoscopically. The weight loss as result of this procedure was initially contributed strictly to restrictive and malabsorption mechanisms. However, in the past few decades we have become aware of the complexity of regulation of the body weight. Obesity is the result of an imbalance in the physiological mechanism that regulates calorie intake and calorie consumption. The complex physiological mechanism is the result assimilation of many complex digestive enzymes and numerous central and peripheral digestive and metabolic hormones and neuro-hormonal pathway as well as gastrointestinal microbial organisms that set our body weight point. Such mechanisms are very powerful and extremely difficult to correct. Thus, weight loss surgery has become a remarkable and an effective and durable tool to correct obesity as well as metabolic disorder and diabetes. The effect of weight loss surgery is more than restriction and malabsorption of food, it is the effect of altering endocrine and neurohormonal effect on metabolically important gastrointestinal microbes that will result in diminished fat storage and changes of behavioral response to perception of hunger and satiety.

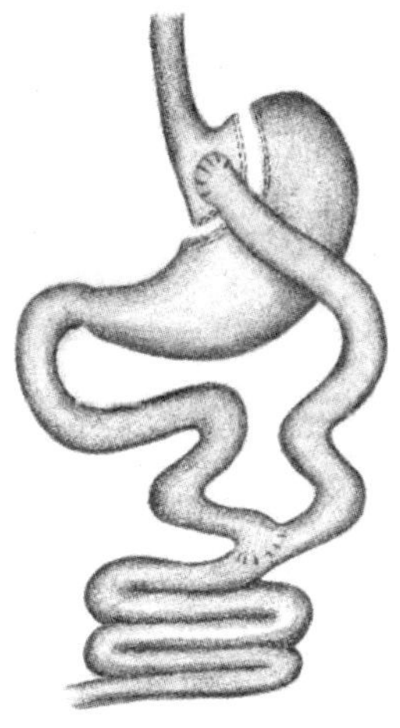

Roux-en-Y gastric bypass

Weight loss surgery is the only established treatment modality for severe obesity with long-term sustainability and effective weight loss. Roux-en-Y gastric bypass by exclusion of passage of food from duodenum eliminates post-prandial secretion of glucagon and glucagon-like hormones. For the same reason the intake of simple carbohydrates and sweets after this procedure will stimulate insulin secretion. However due to lack of insulin resistance (glucagon), there will be a dramatic drop of blood sugar known as dumping syndrome, which exhibits as a profound weakness, sweating, abdominal cramp and diarrhea. Traditionally low blood sugar is treated by sugary drinks; however, such treatment in patients after Roux-en-Y gastric bypass will result in further stimulation of insulin secretion and inevitably drop the blood sugar even lower. Therefore, it is important to know that hypoglycemia (low blood sugar) in post Roux-en-Y gastric bypass patients should not be treated with sugary drinks, it can be reversed by intravenous injection of glucagon. Due to bypass portion of the stomach which aides in the absorption of vitamin B12, after this procedure it is required to take a multivitamin and vitamin B12 supplement to prevent deficiency.

In 1970's multiple gastric weight loss restrictive procedures were introduced as an alternative to gastric bypass such as **horizontal** and **vertical gastroplasty**. In these procedures a partition is created either horizontally or vertically in the upper part of stomach that is connected via a small outlet to the rest of stomach. This procedure became popular in 1980's and 1990's. Even though these procedures had an initial weight loss, over time they had a high level of failure. These procedures are no longer performed as an option for weight loss. There are still some patients that have had gastroplasty that continue experiencing complications or have regained all of their weight back. They require ongoing medical attention and will benefit from revision surgery to eliminate the complications and provide a more effective weight loss procedure.

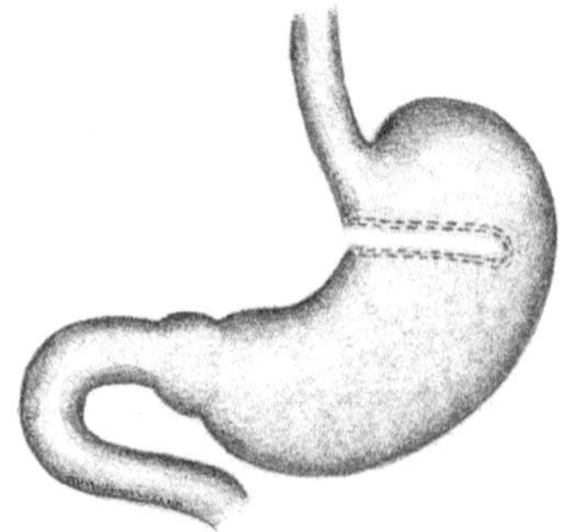

Horizontal gastroplasty

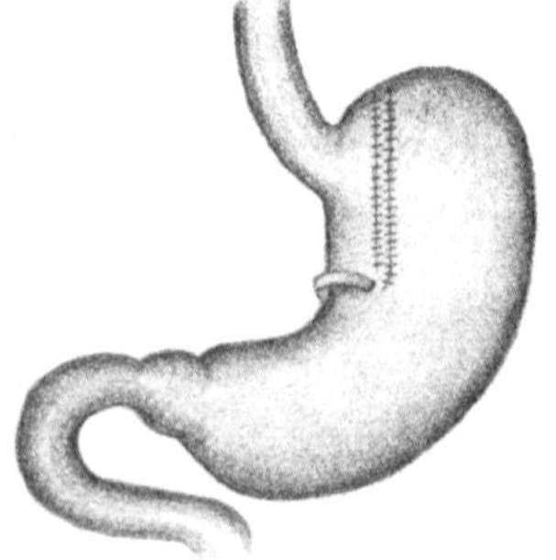

Vertical gastroplasty

In 1978 **gastric banding** with mesh was introduced to divide the stomach into two pouches with a smaller pouch proximal to restrict food intake. This procedure was modified in 1980 as a **Molina band** with use of Dacron or Gore-Tex graft to partition the stomach. The patients who underwent these procedures ultimately developed dilation and failure of procedure. These procedures are no longer being performed. Unfortunately, still there are some patients who have the Molina band in place that have gained their weight back or are experiencing complications from the procedure requiring ongoing medical attention and will benefit from removal of band and revision of the surgery.

In 1983 **adjustable gastric band** was introduced and became popular by 1990. This band is a removable device with an inner inflatable circular cuff of silicon that is placed around the upper part of the stomach that is connected via a tubing to a port placed subcutaneously which can be periodically injected or remove saline to modify the diameter of the band.

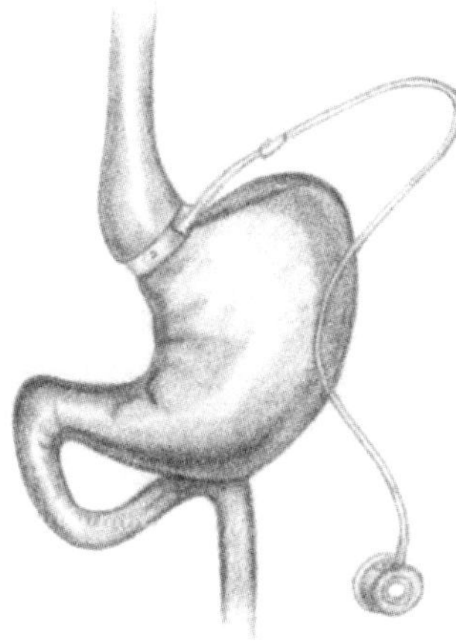

Adjustable gastric band

This procedure is aimed to mechanically restrict food intake, however in reality this concept does not produce any meaningful results. This procedure is now performed laparoscopically with a shortened hospital stay and fast recovery time and has become quite popular. This procedure results in a complication of dilation of the esophagus with reflux of food. Over time this procedure has high rate of failure for weight loss with increased rate of re-operation due to slippage or erosion of band as well as port issues. This procedure has been nearly abandoned as a viable option of weight loss, but still is being performed outside of the United States. There are many patients who still have the band in place and have failed to accomplish any weight loss and they are having complications seeking ongoing medical care that will eventually benefit from removal of band and revisional procedures.

In 1979 **biliopancreatic diversion** was introduced as an alternative to jejunoileal bypass. This procedure has partial small bowel bypassed and partial gastrectomy to combine restrictive procedure with malabsorption. Later on, this procedure was modified to duodenal switch with vertical gastrectomy. These procedures have larger gastric pouches than Roux-en-Y gastric bypass, which allows the patient to eat more but have greater malabsorption component that cause nutritional deficiency of protein, calcium and fat-soluble vitamins. These procedures are currently more popular outside the United States.

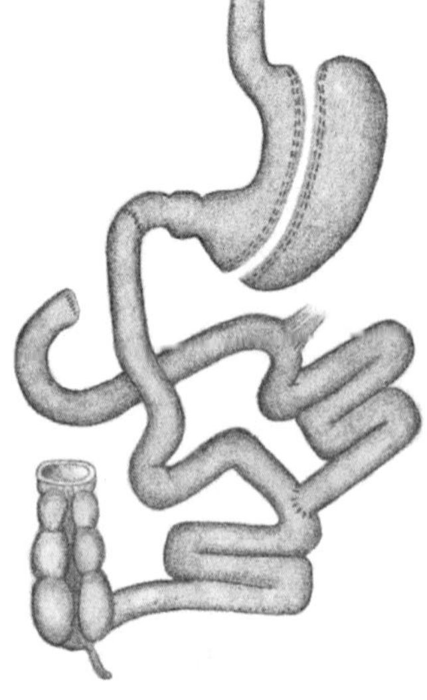

Biliopancreatic diversion

Vertical removal of stomach which is part of biliopancreatic diversion led to development of **sleeve gastrectomy**. This procedure became a viable and an independent weight loss procedure. This procedure is performed laparoscopically. This procedure is not reversible and is performed with staples by removing nearly 80 percent of lateral portion of stomach, from near esophagus to near outlet of stomach (pylorus) and leaving a skinny tubular banana shape stomach. The small stomach gets full quickly with much less food. In addition, as result of the removal of part of the stomach it reduces the secretion of the hormone that causes hunger (Ghrelin) which will result in weight loss.

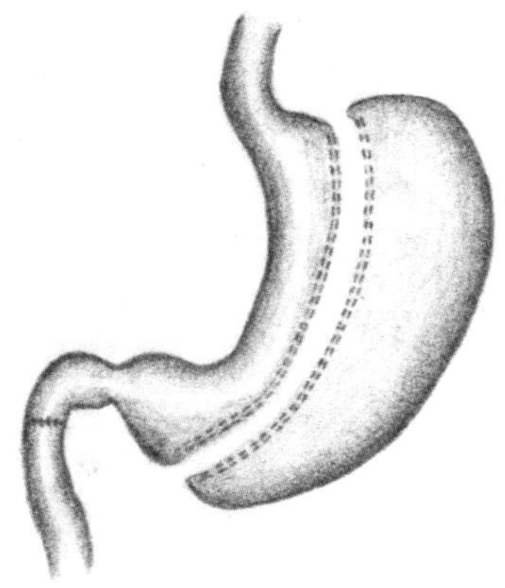

Sleeve gastrectomy

Currently this procedure is the most performed weight loss surgery. Its shortened operative time has made it more attractive in high risk patients or high BMI and if necessary, later on it can be converted to duodenal switch or Roux-en-Y gastric bypass. Acid reflux is the most common complication of this procedure, other complications include stricture, leaks and delay in gastric emptying with chronic nausea and vomiting.

While weight loss surgery remains the most effective treatment for obesity, the quest for safer and less invasive and cost-effective management of obesity has led to development of several less invasive weight loss procedures. These techniques mostly attempt to mimic some of the features of weight loss surgery.

In 1976 **gastric plication** was performed for treatment of obesity. This procedure was performed by dividing vascular attachment of greater curvature of stomach and placing multiple sutures to fold and imbricate greater curvature of stomach and thus reducing the size of stomach. Although this procedure had low complication rate and favorable short-term results it lacked long term weight loss. This procedure later on was performed laparoscopically but still failed to become a viable option for treatment of obesity.

In the recent years endoscopic gastric plication is introduced as **endoscopic sleeve gastrectomy**. This is an incisionless procedure that is performed under general anesthesia with a medical flexible endoscope and endoscopic suturing system. This procedure is performed by placing multiple sutures inside the stomach to reduce the greater curvature of the stomach and reduce the length and width of the gastric cavity to induce weight loss. This procedure is much more limited than laparoscopic gastric plication due to the lack of ability to divide and free the vascular attachment of the greater curvature. Additionally, suturing the wall of the stomach from inside of the stomach will result in poor healing and fusion of the gastric wall. Sooner or later the sutures will pull out and the stomach will return to its normal size. This procedure has a very short-term weight loss and is not covered by any insurance providers. The cost is nearly or slightly less than sleeve gastrectomy and has proven not to be cost effective and is hardly a viable option for weight loss.

Intragastric balloon was first introduced in 1985 and it was widely used for treatment of obesity outside of the United States. In 2015 the FDA approved the use of gastric balloon in the United States for treatment of obesity with a BMI less than 30 kg/m^2. It is only approved for 6 months use (short term). Intragastric balloons are used as an alternative to weight loss surgery as a less invasive procedure that is less costly than weight loss surgery, however, the procedure is not covered by most health insurance providers.

Currently 3 different intragastric balloons are approved for the treatment of obesity in the United States.

Orbera is a single fluid filled balloon that is placed under endoscopic guidance and removed in 6 months under endoscopic guidance as well.

ReShape is double balloon fluid filled system that is also placed and removed in 6 months under endoscopic guidance.

Obalon is a one and up to three balloons gas filled system that is placed as a capsule that can be swallowed and placed under radiological guidance without need for endoscopy, however, is removed in 6 months under endoscopic guidance.

The efficacy and long-term results of utilization of gastric balloons has not been established. The mechanism of action of intragastric balloons appear to be through space occupancy of stomach and suppression of Ghrelin and decreased gastric emptying. Ghrelin is a hormone that is secreted from the fundus of the stomach that causes the sensation of hunger and desire to eat. It is speculated that distention and compression of the fundus of the stomach by the balloon causes reduction of the secretion of the Ghrelin hormone. However, after removal of gastric balloon gastric emptying and Ghrelin secretion quickly return to normal levels and then leads to significant weight gain after the balloon has been removed.

Intragastric balloons are becoming increasingly popular as an alternative for weight loss surgery specifically in individuals who are afraid of surgery. However, intragastric balloons have a poor safety profile and studies have shown that intragastric balloon have twice the adverse outcome than weight loss surgery. Complications such as intolerance of balloon requiring early removal, gastric outlet obstruction, intestinal obstruction due to migration of spontaneous deflation of balloon, gastric ulcer and gastric perforation. In 2017 FDA issued an alert after five unanticipated deaths were reported following use of gastric balloons. Due to the temporary effect of the intragastric balloons and the high rate of unanticipated adverse effects which includes morbidity, this modality of treatment will hardly count as a viable solution for treatment of obesity.

Vagal blockade. Vagus nerve plays a significant role in regulating stomach function. Vagal block system placement is minimally invasive, and it includes two electrodes that are placed laparoscopically on the anterior and posterior of Vagus nerve near the junction of stomach with esophagus. These electrodes are connected to a rechargeable nerve regulator that is placed in a pocket under the skin in the chest area. This unit delivers signals for 12 hours a day that filters signals from Vagus nerve and blocks the connection between stomach and brain (hypothalamus) to suppress appetite. The device is removable and is charged for 60-90 minutes twice a week. This device was approved by FDA as a weight loss option, but currently the device and its surgical implementation is not covered by any insurance carrier and its cost exceeds the cost of sleeve gastrectomy or Roux-en-Y gastric bypass.

The experience with Roux-en-Y gastric bypass has shown that exclusion of passage of food from duodenum and small bowel plays an important role in reducing insulin resistance and reducing blood sugar and enhancing weight loss. This has led to development of **EndoBarrier**, which is an endoscopic Duodenal-Jejunal Bypass Liner (DJBL); which is an endoscopic device placed under radiological control. It is a 62 cm thin plastic sleeve with a proximal part for fixation in duodenum. It prevents contact of food with duodenum and proximal small bowel and impedes contact of food with bile and pancreatic enzymes. EndoBarrier is a possibility for treatment of obesity and Type 2 diabetes mellitus. The device is still under experimentation and needs improvement before being approved for use in the United States.

AspireAssist is the endoscopic assisted percutaneous placement of a tube into the stomach. Once it's healed it can be connected to aspiration system to aspirate approximately 30 percent of ingested food thus reducing calorie intake. This procedure does not alter any metabolic or induce any physiological change in the body. It encourages overconsumption of food intake and will not promote lifestyle changes.

* * *

It has been nearly five decades since surgery was introduced in the treatment of obesity. In the early days weight loss surgery was performed by an open technique. It wasn't until three decades ago that minimally invasive laparoscopic surgery was introduced in the treatment of obesity. Enhanced recovery from laparoscopic surgery, markedly diminished post-op pain and practically eliminated post-operative wound problems. Laparoscopy has revolutionized the surgical treatment of obesity.

Artificial intelligence and computer technology in recent years has brought a new frontier to the surgeons' laparoscopic skills in the surgical treatment of obesity. Computer assisted robotic surgery has revolutionized bariatric surgery. It has added more flexibility and precision to these procedures. Robotic bariatric surgery holds a promising future for weight loss surgery particularly for complex weight loss surgical procedures and those requiring revision of previous weight loss surgery.

Revision of adjustable gastric banding. Gastric banding is proven to be associated with a high rate of failure of weight loss with increased rate of complications. Many patients will benefit from removal of the band and the performance of a more effective weight loss surgery such as sleeve gastrectomy or Roux-en-Y gastric bypass. In some cases, this conversion can be done in the same setting with the removal of band and port. More often it is preferable to remove the band and allow stomach to heal and perform secondary procedure at a later date to avoid complications such as failure of the staple line to heal and/or leak.

In the case of perforation of the band in the stomach it is preferable that laparoscopically remove the band from inside the stomach (trans gastric) to avoid leakage of gastric contents of stomach into the abdominal cavity. After proper healing and recovery from the procedure a secondary weight loss procedure can be performed at a later date.

Revision of vertical banded gastroplasty. This procedure was popular in the 1980's and 1990's. Even though this procedure is no longer performed, there are still some patients that have had this procedure and regained all or most of their weight. Many of them are suffering from complications associated with the procedure. These patients will benefit from conversion to sleeve gastrectomy or Roux-en-Y gastric bypass. However, depending on the degree of difficulty of taking down adhesions (scar tissue) and extensive deformity of stomach it may be advisable to separate the existing staple line by laparoscopically entering inside the stomach and use staples to divide old staple line to convert stomach to one cavity (trans-gastric gastro-gastrostomy) and later can convert the procedure to a sleeve gastrectomy or Roux-en-Y gastric bypass.

Revision of Molina band. This procedure was popular in 1980's and 1990's. Patients whom have the Molina band that have gained their weight back or are having difficulty keeping their food down need revision. Some of bands that were placed with Dacron and the stomach tissue has grown into it, the band cannot be removed through laparoscopy from outside of the stomach. These bands can be removed from inside of the stomach endoscopically by placement of a self-expanding stent to force complete perforation of band into stomach cavity and then removal of band with endoscopy after 2-3 weeks.

Revision of sleeve gastrectomy. Failure of adequate weight loss or gaining the initial weight loss a few years after a sleeve gastrectomy may occur. This is due to the genetic predisposition of obesity that over time will reverse the metabolic changes that the sleeve gastrectomy has produced. After sleeve gastrectomy the Ghrelin hormone that is secreted from fundus of stomach will be significantly diminish. This hormone causes hunger and desire to eat, however over a period of time stomach will adapt to this change and begin to secrete Ghrelin during fasting which causes an increase in appetite and weight gain. There is also a gradual expansion and stretching of the stomach a few years after the surgery, that results in being able to eat substantially more food in one setting. Overtime this may lead to returning to faulty eating habits similar to prior weight loss surgery. If there is a substantial increase in the size of the stomach after sleeve gastrectomy a redo sleeve will be beneficial. Otherwise converting sleeve gastrectomy to Roux-en-Y gastric bypass or duodenal switch will be the option of treatment.

Revision of Roux-en-Y gastric bypass. A gradual stretching and expansion of gastric pouch and its outlet to small bowel can occur a few years after Roux-en-Y gastric bypass. This results in increased appetite and ability to eat substantially more food in one setting and weight gain. Using endoscopic suturing and reducing off the size of the pouch and its outlet has shown to be effective to restore proper eating habits and continued weight loss. Aside from restrictive part of Gastric bypass, exclusion of passage of food from duodenum induces metabolic changes that contribute to weight loss. Genetic predisposition of obesity overtime will reverse the metabolic changes induced by Roux-en-Y gastric bypass and restore it to preoperative stage that will result in increased appetite, over drive to eat and weight gain. Revision of Roux-en-Y gastric bypass can be accomplished via laparoscopy or robotic surgery to reduce the size of the gastric pouch and prolong the length of Roux limb to decrease food intake and promote less absorption of calories.

* * *

Chapter 16
Treatment of childhood and adolescent obesity

Children who suffer from obesity are at a significant disadvantage. Prevention of obesity in childhood and adolescent is the key factor, because once obesity occurs, effective treatment is very difficult. Invariably to address an effective plan of treatment requires a multidisciplinary system with clinical psychologist, social worker, dietitian, physicians and surgeon.

Aside from genetic predisposition, in many cases, youth obesity is associated with habitual and misguided eating disorders. The most common type of eating disorder seen in youth obesity is binge eating, loss of control of eating with frequent grazing and night eating syndrome. Contributing factors to adolescent and childhood obesity are faulty dynamics of household. Parental obesity and history of child maltreatment such as emotion, physical or sexual abuse. These are challenging issues that require proper evaluation and appropriate therapy. Youth alcohol or drug misuse must not be overlooked. Behavioral modification such as proper eating habits and exercise as well as multidisciplinary approach need to be implemented and **surgical treatment should not be considered as last resort.**

Development of comorbid condition such as cardiovascular disease, hypertension, type II diabetes, fatty infiltration of liver, idiopathic intracranial hypertension, sleep apnea, gastroesophageal reflux disease and orthopedic complications of obesity are strong consideration for weight loss surgery. Children of ages 10-19 with any comorbid conditions or severe obesity causing significant impairment of quality of life should be strongly considered for surgical weight loss treatment. State of bone growth and psychological or social conditions are not any contraindication to surgical treatment.

Considering maturity of the child, both parents and child should be informed of risk and benefit of surgery and long-term outcome. They must understand lifelong commitment for vitamin intake, life style modification, increased physical activity and follow up.

Although multiple surgical treatments have been advocated for treatment of adolescent obesity, sleeve gastrectomy is preferred choice of weight loss surgery for such population. This procedure is considered to be safe and effective treatment of severe obesity in adolescents.

Adjustable gastric banding due to its poor weight loss result and high risk of complication and requiring reoperation is not recommended for adolescent or even adult weight loss surgery.

Although Roux-en-Y gastric bypass is the most efficient and durable treatment for obesity, it should not be considered as the primary weight loss treatment of adolescent obesity. This procedure can be considered as a secondary option of treatment in case of future failure of weight loss after sleeve gastrectomy few years down the road.

Biliopancreatic diversion due to high complication of surgery and malabsorption is not considered for adolescent weight loss surgery.

Anti-obesity medications have limited effect in treatment of childhood and adolescent obesity. These medications have temporary effect and have high rate of adverse effect, they are used as adjuvant treatment with life style changes and surgical treatment.

Orlistat (Alli)

Is the most common medication that is being approved to be used in adolescent of ages 12-16 (see chapter 14).

Other medications such as topiramate, metformin and fluoxetine are used in treatment of adolescent obesity (see chapter 14).

Use of FDA approved alternative emerged technology for adults such as intragastric balloon, vagal stimulator and gastric aspiration devices are not recommended in children and adolescent treatment of obesity. These procedures lack durability and only should be considered if standard procedures are unavailable.

* * *

Chapter 17

Nutritional guideline following weight loss surgery

It is best to start a full liquid diet at least a week prior to the weight loss or metabolic surgery. It is recommended to start a multivitamin supplement prior to the surgery. All the herbal supplements should be discontinued for at least a week or 10 days prior to surgery. Anti-inflammatory medication, arthritis medication and aspirin should be stopped a week prior to the surgery. Antiplatelet medication and oral anticoagulation must be stopped under discretion of physician and if necessary injectable subcutaneous anticoagulation will be prescribed by your physician. You must discuss with your physician about preoperative directions regarding whether to take or not your high blood pressure or diabetic medication on the day of surgery.

You can have full liquid up to 6 hours before the surgery and clear liquid up to 4 hours before surgery. After surgery when you leave the hospital follow your doctor's guidance regarding your medications and anticoagulant (blood thinner). Your doctor may give you other directions to follow, always follow your doctor's advice.

Generally, post weight loss and metabolic surgery patients follow the Stage I diet for a week. The purpose of this diet is to allow surgically altered stomach to heal.

Stage I diet is a clear liquid diet that consists of water (can add crystal light), sugar free popsicles, sugar free gelatin, beef or chicken broth or bouillon, decaffeinated tea or coffee. You may add artificial sweetener. Avoid carbonated drinks, no sugary or alcoholic beverages. Drinking liquid and water in is the most important nutrient for our body, it plays a key role in the digestion, absorption and transporting nutrients, make sure you are sipping on clear liquid or water throughout the day and drink as much as you tolerate otherwise you can easily become dehydrated. If you are not emptying your bladder at least 3 times a day you are not getting enough fluids. This is very important for the first few weeks after surgery. Check the color of your urine it should be pale yellow, if it is dark yellow you are not drinking enough clear liquids.

After one week you will start on Stage II diet for 2 to 3 weeks this diet is full liquid diet you can still take all clear liquids, skim milk, low fat cream and soups (strain with wire mesh), sugar free pudding, smooth lite yogurt (non-fat, not sweetened), low fat cottage cheese and runny eggs. No juices, no sugary drinks, no sodas and no protein shakes.

Three to four weeks after surgery you will advance to Stage III diet. This is low fat low carb soft diet, soft scrambled eggs, egg beaters, low fat cottage cheese, water packed tuna, caned fish, baked soft fish, sliced thin deli turkey or chicken, soft low-fat cheese and soft mashed cooked beans. At this stage separate food and liquid by 30 minutes, you only eat 3 times a day, no smoking, may drink liquids between the meals, no carbs, no mashed potatoes, no pasta, no protein shakes. As appropriated in 4 to 6 weeks after surgery advance to high protein regular food as you can tolerate.

It is important to take vitamin and mineral supplements after weight loss and metabolic surgery as recommended.

Multivitamin. One week after surgery, start chewable or liquid multivitamin, twice a day.

Calcium. Three to four weeks after surgery start chewable calcium citrate individual dose take 1200-1500 mg daily. Separate your calcium and multivitamin supplement by at least two hours.

Iron. Make sure that your multivitamin supplement is complete and contain some iron. Women of childbearing age (premenopausal) are at increased risk of developing iron deficiency and anemia. It is recommended to take additional iron supplement 3-

4 weeks after weight loss and metabolic surgery, it is important to take 1 mg of folic acid in addition to iron daily.

Vitamin B12. It is recommended to take 250-500 mg B12 daily, it can be in form of tablet, liquid, nasal spray or injectable.

Thiamine. This vitamin has a short half-life after weight loss surgery, 10-20 days of lack of adequate nutrition can cause thiamine deficiency. In addition, the use of commonly prescribed medication after weight loss surgery like Zantac, Pepcid or Nexium and some diuretics such as Lasix can interfere with the absorption of thiamine. In order to prevent thiamine deficiency post-surgery that can contribute to nausea and anorexia, it is recommended to take 100 mg of thiamine daily.

* * *

Our life

We must have dreams in our life because our life is the reflection of our dreams. We must pay the price, work hard, meet the challenges and never quit to make our dreams come true. A dream needs a goal in our life because a dream without a goal is just a dream. We must have a daily goal, a weekly goal, a monthly goal, a yearly goal and above all a life time goal. Life can be tough, but we must find someone to help us through life. We must know that life is not fair, and we will often fail but we must have the will to succeed and never ever give up.

We must discipline ourselves to work hard every day and not to be afraid to go to bed late and still get up early the next day. Little things in life matter, if we can't do the little things right, we won't be able to do the big things right. Start every day with a task and end the day with a task completed and tomorrow will be a better day.

We must respect everyone but first have a sense of self-respect and sense of pride in what we do. We must learn to lift ourselves up but in the meantime lift others up. We must change our life for better, and at the same time the life of others. We must live by each other's happiness.

We must have a positive influence on the lives of others and be the one who inspires them. Remember others will measure us by the size of our hearts and not by who we are. We must understand the meaning of our life. This life is not about what we take when we leave this world; it is about what we leave behind. Remember the future is in our hands. We live the life we choose but the choices we make in our life will have future consequences.

Have a heart that does not hate, have a smile that does not fade and have a touch that does not hurt.

May we have the Lord's mercy and blessing in our lives.

Younan Nowzaradan M.D.